Cooking for Health

Obesity, Weight Loss and Eating Disorders

Macrobiotic Food and Cooking Series

Cooking for Health

Obesity, Weight Loss and Eating Disorders

by Aveline Kushi
edited by Helaine Honig

foreword by Lawrence Haruo Kushi, Sc.D.

Japan Publications, Inc.
Tokyo · New York

Note to the reader: Those with health problems are advised to seek the
guidance of a qualified medical, or psychological professional in addition
to that of a qualized macrobiotic courselor before implementing any of the
dietary and other approaches presented in this book. It is essential that any
reader who has any reason to suspect serious illness in themselves or
their family members seek appropriate medical, nutritional, or psychological advice promptly. Neither this or any other health related book
should be used as a substitute for qualified care or treatment

Published by JAPAN PUBLICATIONS, INC , Tokyo and New York

Distributors:
UNITED STATES: *Kodansha International/USA, Ltd., through Harper & Row,
Publishers, Inc., 10 East 53rd Street, New York, New York 10022.* SOUTH
AMERICA: *Harper & Row, Publishers, Inc., International Department.*
CANADA: *Fitzhenry & Whiteside Ltd., 195 Allstate Parkway, Markham,
Ontario, L3R 4T8.* MEXICO AND CENTRAL AMERICA: *HARLA S. A. de C. V.,
Apartado 30–546, Mexico 4, D. F.* BRITISH ISLES: *International Book Dis-
tributors Ltd., 66 Wood Lane End, Hemel Hempstead, Herts HP2 4RG.*
EUROPEAN CONTINENT: *Fleetbooks, S. A., c/o Feffer and Simons (Nederland)
V. V., Rijnkade 170, 1382 GT Weesp, The Netherlands.* AUSTRALIA AND
NEW ZEALAND: *Bookwise International, 1 Jeanes Street, Beverley, South
Australia 5007.* THE FAR EAST AND JAPAN: *Japan Publications Trading
Co., Ltd., 1–2–1, Sarugaku-cho, Chiyoda-ku, Tokyo 101.*

First edition: June 1987

LCCC No. 85–081369
ISBN 0–87040–642–6

Printed in U.S.A.

Foreword

This volume of the *Macrobiotic Food and Cooking Series* focuses on obesity, a condition many nutritionists agree is the major food-related disorder in the United States today. Certainly, overweight is a risk factor for the major causes of death and disability—it contributes to heart disease, several types of cancer, and diabetes.

If obesity is one extreme on a spectrum of eating disorders, anrexia nervosa and bulimia are, in the United States, the other extreme. Yet, as is frequently the case, the two extremes are often products of similar circumstances. Thus, we come to appreciate the paradox that results in anorexia and bulimia reaching epidemic proportion in our society, while overweight is a major physical and social problem.

It is generally acknowledged that two major factors contribute to obesity in the United States. The first is the sedentary lifestyle we have adapted over the past several decades. We use microwave ovens to heat our pre-packaged meals; our automobiles take us from our front door to our work place; and we ride elevators and escalators instead of using the stairs. Many of us must make a concerted effort to physically challenge ourselves by scheduling time at our local fitness club.

Contrast this lifestyle with that of our grandparents and great-grandparents, who probably were farmers or who could at least relate to gardening and agriculture. They probably engaged in more physical activity in their daily lives than we manage to schedule into ours. Thus, even though we eat less per capita now than we did at the turn of the century, we also weigh more.

The second major factor that contributes to obesity in our society is the excess fat in the diet of most Americans. It is the nature of foodstuffs that, gram for gram, fat contains more energy than either protein or carbohydrate. Other things being equal, a high-fat diet thus leads to consumption of more calories and the need to store more calories in the form of body fat.

At the same time that we are faced with a diet that promotes weight gain and a lifestyle that discourages weight loss, we are confronted with societal ideals of body shape that promote figures far slimmer than was the ideal just several decades ago. Not suprisingly, we are forced into a situation where extreme attempts to attain ideal body shapes turn into potentially devastating eating disorders.

The practical suggestions in this book, along with the insights contained in the companion volume, *The Macrobiotic Health Education Series*, will give readers a comprehensive understanding of eating disorders. The two volumes can lead one to a healthier body, mind, and spirit.

Lawrence Haruo Kushi, Sc.D.
Minneapolis, Minnesota,
December, 1986

Acknowledgments ━━━━━━━━

I would like to thank all of our friends who assisted in completing this volume. I thank our friend and associate, Helaine Honig, for compling and editing the materials, and extend appreciation to Jay Kelly and Lilian Kushi for contributing the illustrations and artwork.

I thank our associates, Edward and Wendy Esko, for their guidance and support, and thank the friends who assisted Michio Kushi in completing the companion volume in the *Macrobiotic Health Education Series, Obesity, Weight Loss, and Eating Disorders,* including John David Mann, the editor of the book.

I extend my appreciation to Iwao Yoshizaki and Yoshiro Fujiwara, respectively president and American representative of Japan Publications, Inc., for their guidance and advice, and thank my son, Lawrence Haruo Kushi, for writing the Foreword to this volume. Finally, I thank our friend Phillip Jannetta, currently living in Tokyo, for doing the editorial work on this book.

Contents

1. Underlying Cosmology ━━━

There is a vast cosmology behind the principles of macrobiotics,
a cosmology which sets out to explain the creation and the interrelationship of all phenomena throughout the universe.

The real purpose of macrobiotics is to empower us with the ability
to fulfill our potentials and dreams, and to serve as a reminder that
we are the builders and masters of our own lives.

Macrobiotics is a rich and unlimited field of study that extends far
beyond the scope of this book. Readers are encouraged to investigate
the infinite applications of the macrobiotic principles, which are also
called the Unifying Principles. In doing so, individuals can become
their own guide, discovering for themselves what is needed to maintain health and to accomplish personal goals. This chapter contains
a brief overview of the macrobiotic principles and how they apply to
the particular subjects of diet and health. For more detailed information, and for examples of applying the Unifying Principles to other
areas, readers are referred to any of the variety of books listed in the
bibliography.

Everything in the universe is a constantly moving and changing
energy, varying in density and speed. Even seemingly stable and solid
objects, a rock or a table for instance, are made up of moving molecules, atoms, electrons and protons, which themselves are nothing but
energy.

The origin and destination of all phenomena is Infinity, also called
God, the Universal Will, the Super Consciousness, or Nothingness.
There is no time or space, past or future, light or darkness here.
There is only endless motion, moving at an infinite speed in all directions.

These currents of endless motion (refer to Fig. 1) intersect and
create logarithmic spirals which spin inwards towards the center in
a contracting, centripetal direction (also referred to as the *yang* force).
At their most contracted point, these inward-moving spirals reverse
direction to create opposite logarithmic spirals which spin outwards
from the center in an expanding, centrifugal direction (also referred
to as the *yin* force). The formation of these spirals is the means by
which everything comes into being and eventually dissolves. In fact,

these opposite and complementary forces, by their constant interaction, are creating all things, material and non-material. Figure 1 (reprinted from the *Book of Do-In: Exercise for Physical and Spiritual Development* by Michio Kushi, p. 18) shows the "Eternal and Universal Cycle of Change."

When moving in a yang (△) direction, energy begins to take on form in a process of materialization. Generally speaking, this process is characterized by increasing speed, increasing temperature, and more density and weight which manifest as compactness or contraction.

Fig. 1   The Eternal and Universal Cycle of Change

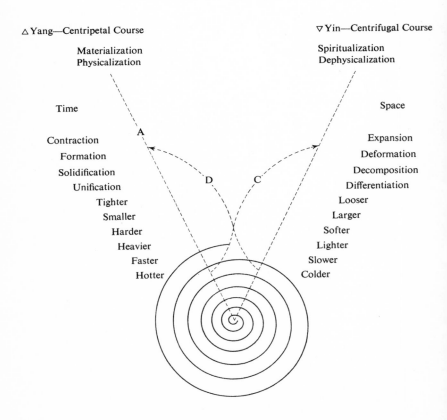

△ Yang—Centripetal Course

Materialization
Physicalization

Time

Contraction
Formation
Solidification
Unification
Tighter
Smaller
Harder
Heavier
Faster
Hotter

∇ Yin—Centrifugal Course

Spiritualization
Dephysicalization

Space

Expansion
Deformation
Decomposition
Differentiation
Looser
Larger
Softer
Lighter
Slower
Colder

When moving in a yin (∇) direction, energy takes on the opposite characteristics. It is slower, cooler, more diffused, expanded, and lighter in weight. Yang motion is followed by yin, and yin motion is followed by yang. Yang does not exist without yin, nor yin without yang.

Fig. 2   The Creation of the Universe

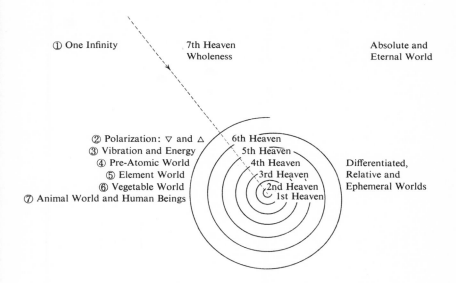

① One Infinity   7th Heaven Wholeness   Absolute and Eternal World

② Polarization: ∇ and △
③ Vibration and Energy
④ Pre-Atomic World
⑤ Element World
⑥ Vegetable World
⑦ Animal World and Human Beings

6th Heaven
5th Heaven
4th Heaven
3rd Heaven
2nd Heaven
1st Heaven

Differentiated, Relative and Ephemeral Worlds

① *One Infinity:*   Absolute and eternal; nothing but infinite motion.
② *Polarization— Yin (∇) and Yang (△):*   The beginning of time and space, direction, dimensions, relativity, differentiation, and the ephemeral world.
③ *Vibration and Energy:*   The beginning of light, sound, long and short waves, the subconscious and conscious mind, mental and spiritual phenomena.
④ *Pre-Atomic World:*   The world of electrons, neutrons, and other pre-atomic particles, and the beginning of the material world.
⑤ *Elemental World:*   The world of molecules, the elements (hydrogen, helium, etc.), soil, water, air, fire, our senses, and the beginning of the visible world.
⑥ *Vegetable World:*   The plant kingdom.
⑦ *Animal World and Human Beings:*   The animal kingdom, including human beings.

All phenomena are created from these two opposite forces or directions of yin and yang which, in turn, grew out of what we call God, Infinity, and so on. Figure 2 is a spirallic illustration of the "Creation of the Universe." (Reprinted from the *Book of Do-In* by Michio Kushi, p. 23.)

Human beings, as the end result of a yang, centripetal spiral, are also at the beginning of a yin, centrifugal spiral. As we develop in a more yang direction, we are created by physical food, the elemental energies from the sun, water, wind, and so on, and the vibrations of thoughts from the mind. After we are formed in the physical world, we start to grow in the opposite, or yin direction, as we develop emotionally, mentally, and spiritually. Eventually, our physical body decomposes and our soul or consciousness continues to develop towards its ultimate merging with Infinity itself.

Fig. 3   The Eternal Cycle of Life

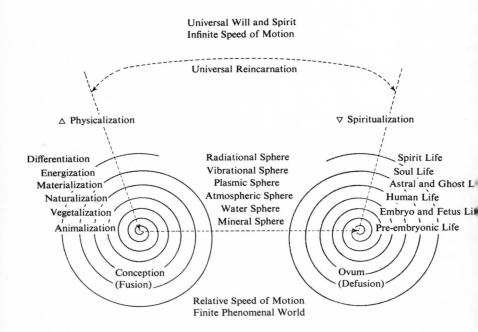

Figure 3 shows the "Eternal Cycle of Life." (Reprinted from the *Book of Do-In* by Michio Kushi, p. 33.)

As illustrated, the most contracted or yang point, the fusion of sperm and egg, is immediately followed by the yin, expanding force reflected in the rapid cell division of the fertilized egg. (Yang, at its extreme point, turns into yin, and vice versa.) This is followed by pre-embryonic life, and then the watery and totally dark world of the embryo and fetus. At birth, we begin life in the airy atmosphere of our human environment. This world of air is half in darkness and half in light. When we pass away, we shed our physical body and enter the plasmic, astral world of ghosts or spiritual phenomena, which is totally immersed in light. Each of the above successive worlds becomes progressively more expansive, freer, and involves a longer so-called time span.

By maintaining a healthy mind, body, and spirit, we are able to move more smoothly and happily into the next world. A pregnant woman has traditionally been advised to get proper and balanced nourishment, sufficient exercise and rest, and to avoid violence in pastimes—movies, books, and the like. She is also advised to send happy and beautiful thoughts to the baby so that the infant can come into this world in a healthy, happy state. In this way the child can live more peacefully and unencumbered. Likewise, in this life, we can all consider the quality of the various types of food we receive, the kinds of exercise and physical activity and rest we take, and in general, reflect on our entire way of life. In addition, we can encourage positive, creative thoughts and actions so that our birth into the next world will be smooth and our life there will be unimpeded.

The spirits of unhappy persons are full of sorrow and delusion, and instead of moving forward and onward into a brighter, freer world of light, they remain attached to the earthly level and to the people and places they knew. The Oriental and other "primitive" cultures send their consolation, love, and wishes of happiness to their deceased ancestors. This helps to free these spirits and assists their ascent onto a broader and more joyful plane of existence.

We are all traveling back towards the outer parts of the universal spiral of life as we search for freedom, peace of mind, happiness, the ability to spread our wings and, finally, to be one with God. Even those who seemingly want only money or possessions are actually looking for this same happiness and freedom and they feel it will result from their material pursuits. It is proper that each person pursues what he or she feels is important at a given point. This is our freedom.

Paradoxically, as many religions teach, we already are where we want to be. We, as individuals, are a miniature version of the whole universe. Deep inside, each of us knows that there is a larger I or self, a part of us that is eternal, all-knowing, and subject to no boundaries. There is a more synchronized feeling of unity, oneness, and connection between our smaller I, our human existence, and our larger I, this infinite universe, when we are in a relaxed, healthy, vibrant, in-tune-with-nature state. We can tap into the unlimited, creative potential that we have in the universe and use it to direct our life with much more awareness when we are in harmonious synchronicity.

The deeper meaning of health is being in this aligned and synchronous state which results in a smooth, unblocked, effortless flow of our energies between all the inner and outer universal parts of ourselves. The macrobiotic approach to well-being is a holistic approach directed by our understanding that a change in any aspect or portion of our body or self has an effect on everything else including the world and the universe. There are several approaches one can take to create a free flow of energy:

1. *Dietary changes:* Making dietary changes is the major focus of this book. What we eat creates our blood cells, and hence fundamentally influences the formation of organs and all other parts of our body. Although recognition is slowly emerging, it is a wonder that food is not more often identified as a major cause of disease. One's diet also alters the mind and emotions. We know that the ingestion of alcohol and various licit and illicit drugs affects one's mental state. This fact cannot be argued. Likewise, anything that we take in has its affect on our being, though it may be on a subtle level.

2. *Working with the powers of the mind:* Everything that exists has its origin in the invisible world of the mind and vibrations. It is said that what we believe manifests. There are many negative thoughts or assumptions that we may dwell on which can influence our lives. Many of these delusions as we may call them occur automatically and unconsciously. One may develop self-awareness by constantly observing the thoughts, actions, and reactions that control one's life, and make meaningful changes by rechanneling unwanted habits into more positive ideas and dreams.

3. *Relaxation:* Mental and physical tension block the freest flow of energy. A technique one may try is to take an inventory of all the parts of your body and then to relax all tense spots. The same practice can be done with the mind, letting go of anxiety, guilt, and anger. Use the breath to help the relaxation process: breathe slowly and deeply.

4. *Ki-energy related practices:* Palm-healing, shiatsu massage, moxibustion, acupuncture, chiropractics, and others can be used to temporarily unblock stagnations of energy in the body.

5. *Keeping mentally and physically active:* Exercise, do sports, dance, clean house, garden, read, study, engage in hobbies, draw, write, compose, play music, do volunteer work, teach . . . whatever seems appealing. Make sure to do both mental and physical work. The more energy we circulate, the more comes back to us, and the less stagnation there is in our lives.

6. *Changing one's environmental surroundings:* In some cases, it might be necessary to change one's environmental surroundings. Some forms of sickness can be more easily eliminated in a warm climate while others may require cooler temperatures. Moving to a quieter locale may be beneficial for some conditions. Also, it is important that one be in a loving atmosphere with people who care about us and support us. We can help maintain a clean, ecologically balanced environment by using biodegradable products and materials, by not taking more than we need, and by helping to protect the well-being of our fellow inhabitants on this earth—the members of the plant and animal kingdoms.

7. *Maintaining good relations with all the people in our lives:* Blaming, holding grudges, anger, fear and hatred make one very tense and cause blockages. We create the circumstances of our individual lives so it is up to us to change them. Give everyone your love, support, and respect for their freedom and individuality.

8. *Being grateful for all that we have been given:* Notice all the beauty and marvels in the world. Look at hardships, difficulties, or rejections as opportunities for self-reflection and growth.

Working on just one of the above recommendations can be tremendously helpful and have a positive effect on us overall. However, to make a really permanent and thorough change for the better, all of the above should be worked on, as they are interrelated. Many people form an exclusive allegiance to one approach and as time passes they wonder why their plans and dreams do not progress beyond a certain point. They then abandon their practice and either give up or make an exclusive attachment to another approach. Please be aware of this tendency and use all the dimensions of your daily life for personal growth.

Yin and Yang

Everything is created and governed by the interactions of yin and yang, the two opposite poles which are endlessly manifesting in the world. The chart on page 19 lists some classification examples.

By learning how yin and yang relate to each other, we can begin to understand the workings of life itself. Civilization's greatest teachings—moral, philosophical, and religious—reveal the interplay of these two primary forces. Macrobiotic dietary recommendations are based on the principles that govern these fundamental forces. The Unifying Principles of macrobiotics can be summarized briefly as follows.

1. *Yin attracts yang and yang attracts yin.* This results in the harmony and marriage of opposites. Examples include man and woman; plus and minus magnets or electrical charges; electron and proton; spirit and matter; and so on. Upon ingesting a quantity of salt (yang) for instance, one is attracted to liquids (yin).

2. *Yin repels yin, and yang repels yang.* For example, oil and water do not mix. Both are yin. Also, two plus poles repel each other, as do two minus poles.

3. *The force of attraction (or repulsion) is proportional to the ratio of yin and yang elements.* Their combinations in various proportions create an infinite variety of energies and phenomena where no two things are identical.

4. *Yin and yang are in constant motion.* They are always flowing from one to another in various degress. Yin in the extreme changes

to yang and vice versa. Nothing is static, and nothing lasts forever. Day turns to night, and night back to day. Activity is followed by rest, rest by activity. Success follows failure and failure follows success. Civilizations rise and fall. What has a beginning has an end.

Attribute	Yin/Centrifugal (▽)	Yang/Centripetal(△)
Tendency	Expansion	Contraction
Function	Dispersion, decomposition	Assimilation, organization
Movement	More inactive, slower	More active, faster
Vibration	Shorter waves, high frequency	Longer waves, low frequency
Direction	Vertical, ascending	Horizontal, descending
Position	More outward and peripheral	More inward and central
Weight	Lighter	Heavier
Temperature	Colder	Hotter
Light	Darker	Lighter
Humidity	More wet	More dry
Density	Thinner	Thicker
Size	Larger	Smaller
Shape	More expanded, fragile	More contracted, harder
Length	Longer	Shorter
Texture	Softer	Harder
Atomic particle	Electron	Proton
Elements	N, O, K, P, Ca	H, C, Na, As, Mg
Environment	Vibration→Air→Water→	Earth
Climate	Tropical	Arctic
Biology	Vegetable	Animal
Sex	Female	Male
Organ structure	Hollow, expansive	Compact, condensed
Nerves	Orthosympathetic	Parasympathetic
Attitude	Gentle, negative	Active, positive
Work	Psychological & mental	Physical & social
Consciousness	More universal	More specific
Mental function	Dealing with the future	Dealing with the past
Culture	Spiritually oriented	Materially oriented
Color	Purple→Blue→Green→Yellow→	Brown→Orange→Red
Season	Winter	Summer
Dimension	Space	Time
Taste	Hot→sour→sweet→	Salty→Bitter
Vitamins	C	K, D
Catalyst	Water	Fire

5. *Nothing is totally yin or totally yang.* All things are made up of both. The more yin something is, the more yang it is as well. Many people that appear yang, strong, rough, and tough on the outside, may in comparision be yin, weak, and fragile on the inside. Those that appear yin, soft, and fragile on the outside may well be yang, strong, and stubborn on the inside.

   Something that is structurally yang, as is the dense and compact body-organ, the liver, is energetically yin; it functions without much motion. Something that is structurally yin, as is the hollow body-organ, the heart, is energetically more yang; it never stops pumping, contracting and expanding. The bigger the front, the bigger the back.

6. *Large yin attracts small yin, large yang attracts small yang.* After consuming sugar (large yin) we are drawn to drink more fluids (small yin).

7. *Yin creates yang, yang creates yin.* A yin, colder climate creates yang, small, hardy vegetation and a more yang, ambitious, hard-driving society. While a yang, warmer climate creates yin, large, lush vegetation and a more slow-paced, easy-going, and relaxed society.

8. *Everything on earth is created by varying proportions of upward and downward energies.* Gravity is an example of downward energy. The growth of trees and plants is an example of upward energy.

Yin and Yang and Diet

Yang foods give warmth, strength, discipline, and vitality. Excessively yang foods (such as red meat, eggs, or too much salt) are known to cause rigidity, egocentricity, exclusivity, restlessness, and violent tendencies on the mental/emotional level, and certain types of cancer and arthritis, for example, on the physical level.

Yin foods are cooling, cleansing, relaxing, and nurture patience and understanding. Excessively yin foods (such as honey, sugar, chemicals and drugs) have been shown to cause weakening and dispersion of the functioning capabilities in body and mind, including fear, defensiveness, loss of will, suspectibility to viruses, a rampage of white-blood-cell production, and depression or suicidal tendencies, to name some common problems.

When taking in overly yang foods, one is automatically attracted to overly yin ones (and vice versa) to make balance and compensation. One may end up on a wild or chaotic seesaw with a combination of unwanted side effects such as the ones listed above. Macrobiotics recommends a diet of more centrally balanced foods. Grains are the most centered and appropriate foods for human beings, requiring only a minimum amount of counterbalancing. (Grains are our complementary opposites as they are the last stage of plant evolution just as we are the last stage of animal evolution.) Brown rice, especially, has the right proportion of yin and yang factors for humans, and provides the most stabilizing dietary staple.

Humans are constitutionally yang, warm-blooded beings and therefore require most if not all of their nourishment from their complementary opposite, which is the yin, vegetable kingdom. Among animal foods, fish is the recommended choice, particularly slow moving, white-meat varieties, as well as some types of shellfish. The human digestive system does not digest or assimilate meat well. It lingers and putrefies in the digestive tract. The only circumstance where it is healthy to eat large amounts of animal food is in the very cold, yin, artic regions where more strongly yang food is needed and where the availability of plant food is minimal.

Actually, climate plays a major role in our choice of available foods. It is recommended that we choose fresh produce which is grown or can grow in our own climatic zone. Tropical fruits are more appropriate when consumed where they are grown. They are detrimental to one's health when taken in large quantities or too often in the temperate zone.

The progression of the seasons also plays an important part in food selection. For instance, in the spring, when the energy is rising and expanding, we should include fresh young greens and sprouts in our meals. Towards fall and then winter, when the energies are descending and contracting, squash, kale, and winter-storable vegetables such as root vegetables, and dried plants such as sea vegetables should be consumed.

A variety of cooking methods should be employed as well. In the winter, we can eat more well-cooked, slightly saltier, pressure-cooked, and baked foods, as well as more fish. In the summer, more lightly cooked, boiled, raw (such as salads and fruits), chilled, and steamed foods and desserts may be consumed.

Also, within one meal we should ideally have a representative variety of cooking styles, as well as a variety of tastes, colors, and sizes.

Two additional factors which determine what is yin and what is yang, and to what relative degree, are: (1) rate of growth (faster is

22

Fig. 4   General Yin (▽) and Yang (△) Categorization of Food

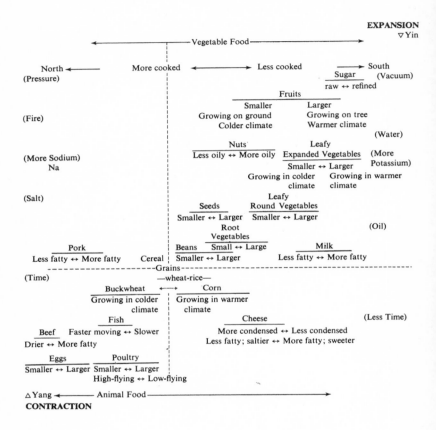

The above chart gives the general classification of food groups from yang to yin. However, more precise classification should be made upon examination of environmental conditions, nature and structure, chemical compounds, and effect upon our physical and mental conditions. Also, cooking can greatly change food qualities from yin to yang and yang to yin.

more yin and slower is more yang), and (2) the portion of the plant being considered—whether roots (more yang) or leaves and fruits (more yin).

Figure 4 represents a general yin/yang categorization of foods. (Reprinted from the *Book of Macrobiotics: The Universal Way of Health and Happiness* by Michio Kushi, p. 57.)

2. Explanation of the Standard Macrobiotic Diet ▬▬▬▬▬▬

These dietary recommendations are suggested for individuals in a generally sound state of health. Persons having a more serious condition may need further modifications. It should also be noted that this is a general guideline and no matter what your condition, each person's individuality, lifestyle and environment need to be taken into account with the diet adapted accordingly.

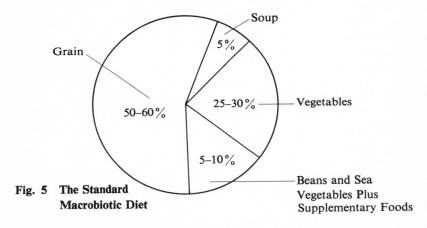

Fig. 5   The Standard Macrobiotic Diet

To see exactly what foods are recommended, refer to the detailed food list following the section below on proportions.

1. WHOLE CEREAL GRAINS.   It is recommended that at least 50 percent of every meal include cooked, organically grown, whole cereal grains prepared in a variety of ways.

2. SOUPS.   Approximately 5 to 10 percent of daily food intake (one or two bowls daily) may include soup made with traditional and naturally processed *miso* or *tamari* soy sauce. The flavor should not be overly salty, and soups may include a variety of grains, beans, and vegetables, including sea vegetables such as *wakame* and *kombu*.

3. VEGETABLES.   About 20 to 30 percent of each meal may include local and organically grown vegetables with a large amount

cooked in various styles and a smaller amount eaten as raw salad.

4. BEANS AND SEA VEGETABLES. Approximately 5 to 10 percent of the daily diet may include cooked beans and sea vegetables.
Sea vegetables may be prepared in a variety of ways. They can
be cooked with beans or vegetables, used in soups, or cooked
and eaten separately as side dishes, flavored with a moderate
amount of tamari soy sauce, sea salt, or rice vinegar.

5. SUPPLEMENTARY FOODS. Foods in the supplementary
category may comprise approximately 5 to 10 percent of a meal.
Once or twice weekly, a small amount of fresh white-meat fish
may be eaten if desired.
Fruit desserts, including fresh and dried fruits, may also be
consumed on occasion. Local and organically grown fruits are
preferred. Frequent use of fruit juice is not advisable. However,
occasional consumption in warmer weather is allowable, depending on our health.
Lightly roasted seeds may be enjoyed as a snack. Though less
frequently, some roasted nuts may be consumed. Rice syrup and
barley malt may be used occasionally to add a sweet taste; rice
vinegar or *umeboshi* vinegar may also be used occasionally for
a sour taste.

6. BEVERAGES. Any traditional tea which does not have an aromatic fragrance or a stimulant effect can be used. Examples
include *bancha* (*kukicha*) twig tea, and roasted grain teas. You
may also drink a moderate amount of water (preferably spring or
well water). Iced drinks are best avoided.

7. FOODS TO BE AVOIDED FOR BETTER HEALTH. Meat,
eggs, animal fat, poultry, dairy products, including butter, yogurt,
ice cream, milk, and cheese.
Tropical or semi-tropical fruits and fruit juices, soda, artificial
drinks and beverages, coffee, colored tea, and all aromatic,
stimulant teas such as mint and peppermint tea.
All artificially colored, preserved, sprayed, or chemically treated
foods. All refined, polished grains, flours, and their derivatives.
Mass-produced industrialized food including all canned and frozen
foods.
Hot spices, any aromatic, stimulant food or food accessory;
artificial vinegar and other seasonings. Licit and illicit drugs are
best avoided. (Medicines prescribed by a physician do not apply

to this general guideline.) Alcohol and cigarettes should be kept to a minimum.

8. ADDITIONAL SUGGESTIONS. Cooking oil should be vegetable quality only. For optimum health, use only cold-pressed, mechanically expelled, unrefined sesame or corn oil in moderate amounts.

Salt should be naturally processed sea salt and excessive use should be avoided. Traditional, non-chemicalized tamari soy sauce and miso may also be used like sea salt.

You may eat regularly two to three times per day, as much as desired, provided the proportion is correct and chewing is thorough (at least 50 times per mouthful or until it becomes liquid). Please avoid eating for approximately three hours before sleeping.

A More Detailed Macrobiotic Food List

Items marked with an asterisk (*) are foods that may have to be avoided or restricted when trying to cure some illnesses; look under the list of diet modifications for specific diseases for more information.

Grains:

Regular use	Occasional use	Occasional flour products
Short-grain brown rice	Long-grain brown rice	Whole wheat noodles*
Medium-grain brown rice	Sweet brown rice	Udon noodles*
Barley	Mochi	Somen noodles*
	Cracked wheat,	Soba noodles (buckwheat)*

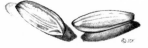

Fig. 6   Short Grain Rice

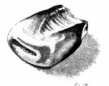

Fig. 8   Dent Corn

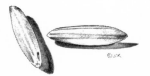

Fig. 7   Bastami Rice

Pearl barley	bulghur	Unyeasted whole
Millet	Steel cut oats	wheat bread*
Corn	Rolled oats*	Unyeasted rye bread*
Corn on the cob	Corn grits*	*Fu**
Whole oats	Corn meal*	*Seitan**
Wheat berries	Rye flakes	
Buckwheat*	Couscous	
Rye		

Vegetables:

Regular use	Occasional use	Avoid
Acorn squash	Celery*	Artichoke
Bok choy	Chives*	Bamboo shoots
Broccoli	Coltsfoot*	Beets
Brussels sprouts	Cucumber*	Curley dock
Burdock	Endive*	Eggplant
Butternut squash	Escarole*	Fennel
Cabbage	Green beans*	Ferns
Carrots & their tops	Green peas*	Ginseng
Cauliflower	Iceberg lettuce*	Green & red peppers
Chinese cabbage	Jerusalem artichoke*	New Zealand spinach
Collard greens	Kohlrabi*	Okra
Daikon & their tops	Lambsquarters*	Plantain
Dandelion roots,	Mushrooms*	Purslane & shepard's
leaves	Patty pan squash*	purse
Hubbard squash	Romaine lettuce*	Potato
Hokkaido pumpkin	Salsify*	Sorrel
Jinenjo	*Shiitake* mushrooms*	Spinach
Kale	Snap beans*	Sweet potato
Leeks	Snow peas*	Swiss chard
Lotus root	Sprouts*	Tomato
Mustard greens	Summer squash*	Taro potato (albi)
Onion	Wax beans*	Yams
Parsley		Zucchini
Parsnip		
Pumpkin		
Radish		
Red cabbage		
Rutabaga		
Scallions		
Turnips & greens		
Watercress		

Beans:

Regular use	Occasional use	Occasional bean substitutes
Azuki beans	Black-eyed peas*	Dried *tofu*
Black soybeans	Black turtle beans*	Fresh tofu*
Chick-peas (garbanzos)	Great northern	*Natto**
Lentils (green)	beans*	*Tempeh**
	Kidney beans*	
	Lima beans*	
	Mung Beans*	
	Navy beans*	
	Pinto beans*	
	Soybeans*	
	Split peas*	
	Whole dried peas*	

Sea Vegetables:

All these sea vegetables can be used regularly. *Arame*, *Hijiki*, Kombu, toasted *Nori*, Wakame, Dulse, Agar-agar, Irish moss, *Mekabu*.

Fruits (usually cooked or dried):

Occasional use	Avoid
Apples*	Avocados
Apricots*	Bananas
Blueberries*	Coconuts
Blackberries*	Dates
Cantaloupes*	Figs
Cherries*	Grapefruit
Grapes*	Kiwi fruit
Lemons (small amounts of juice for cooking)*	Oranges
Peaches*	Mangoes
Pears*	Papayas
Plums*	Persimmons
Raisins*	Pineapple
Raspberries*	All other tropical fruits
Strawberries*	
Watermelon*	

Seeds and Nuts:

Occasional use	Avoid
Almonds*	Brazil nuts
Chestnuts*	Caraway seeds
Peanuts*	Cashews

Pumpkin seeds*	Hazel nuts
Sesame seeds*	Macadamian nuts
Sunflower seeds*	Pistachios
Walnuts*	Poppy seeds
	Spanish peanuts
	All tropical nuts

Animal Foods and Their Products:

Occasional use	Avoid
Carp*	Red-meat fish
Clams*	Chicken
Cod*	All fowl
Flounder*	Eggs
Halibut*	All mammals
Lobster*	All dairy products
Oysters*	
Trout*	
Red snapper*	
Sole*	
White-meat fish in general*	

Pickles:

Regular use	Avoid
Bran pickles	Commercial dill pickles
Brine pickles	Herb pickles
Miso bran pickles	Garlic pickles
Miso pickles	Spiced pickles
Pressed pickles	Apple cider vinegar pickles
Sauerkraut	Wine vinegar pickles
Tamari pickles	
Takuan pickles	

Sweets:

Regular use	Occasional use	Avoid
Cabbage	*Amazake**	All tropical fruits
Carrots	Barley Malt*	Brown sugar
Daikon	Chestnuts*	Carob
Onions	*See* fruit list*	Chocolate
Parsnips	Hot apple cider*	Fructose
Pumpkin	Hot apple juice*	Honey
Squash	Rice malt syrup*	Maple syrup
		Molasses
		White sugar

Beverages:

Regular use	*Occasional use*	*Infrequent use*	*Avoid*
Bancha twig tea (Kukicha)	Grain coffee (100% grain)	Green tea*	Distilled water
Bancha stem tea	Dandelion tea	Vegetable juices*	Coffee
Roasted barley tea	Kombu tea	Juices of fruits from fruit list*	Cold, iced drinks
Roasted brown rice tea	Umeboshi tea	Beer*	Hard liquor
Spring water	*Mu* tea	*Saké*	Herb teas
Well water			Mineral water & all bubbly water
			Regular tea
			Stimulants
			Sugared drinks
			Tap water
			Whiskey
			Wine

Seasonings and Oils:

Regular use	*Occasional use*	*Avoid*
Natural miso	Corn oil*	Animal fats
Dark sesame oil*	Ginger*	Butter & cream
Light sesame oil*	Horseradish*	Coconut oil
Natural soy sauce	*Mirin*	Cottonseed oil
Tamari soy sauce	Olive oil*	Commercial dressings
Unrefined white sea salt	Rice vinegar*	Garlic
Umeboshi plum & paste	Safflower oil*	Linseed oil
Umeboshi vinegar	Sunflower oil*	Margarine
		Mayonnaise
		Commercial miso
		Mustard
		Pepper
		Peanut oil
		Table salt
		All commercial seasonings
		Soybean oil
		Commercial soy sauce
		All spices

Condiments:

Main condiments	*Other condiments*
Gomashio (sesame salt)	Brown rice vinegar
Sea vegetable powder	Cooked miso with scallions &

Sea vegetable powder with
  roasted sesame seeds
Tekka
Umeboshi plum

    onions
    Nori condiment
    Roasted sesame seeds
    Shiso leaves & roasted sesame
      seeds
    Shio Kombu
    Umeboshi plum with raw
      scallions/onions
    Umeboshi vinegar

Snacks:

You can have leftovers, noodles, popcorn (unbuttered), puffed whole cereal grain, rice balls, rice cakes, roasted seeds, *sushi*, and whole wheat bread.

Cooking and Preparation Methods:

Regular use	*Occasional use*
Pressure-cooking	Sautéing*
Boiling	Stir-frying*
Steaming	Raw*
Waterless	Deep-frying*
Soup	*Tempura**
Pickling	Baking*
Oil-less sautéing (with water)	
Pressing	

Cooking Aspects to Change for Variety:

1. Selections of foods within the categories of grains, vegetables, beans, sea vegetables, and so on;
2. Methods of cooking;
3. Ways of cutting vegetables;
4. Amount of water used;
5. Amount and kind of seasoning and condiments used;
6. Length of cooking time;
7. Use of a higher or lower flame;
8. Varying the combination of foods and dishes;
9. Seasonal cooking adjustments.

Way of Life Suggestions and Reminders

- Maintain the dream and image of health, peace, and abundance for yourself, others and the world.
- Live each day happily without being preoccupied with your health, and stay mentally and physically alert and active.

- View everything and everyone you meet with gratitude. Offer thanks before and after each meal.
- It is best to retire before midnight and to get up early in the morning, especially with the sunrise.
- It is best to avoid wearing synthetic or woolen clothing directly against the skin. Wear cotton as much as possible, especially for undergarments. Avoid excessive metallic accessories on the fingers, wrists, or neck. Keep such ornaments simple and graceful.
- If your strength permits, go outdoors in simple clothing. Walk on the grass, beach, or soil up to one half hour every day.
- Keep your home (and other surroundings) in good order, from the kitchen, bathroom, bedroom, living room, to every corner of the house.
- Initiate and maintain an active correspondence, extending best wishes to your family and friends. Also maintain good relationships with everyone around you.
- Avoid taking long hot baths or showers unless you have been consuming too much salt or animal food.
- Scrub your entire body with a hot, damp towel until the skin becomes red, every morning or every night before retiring. If that is not possible, at least scrub your hands, feet, fingers and toes.
- Avoid chemically perfumed cosmetics. For care of the teeth, brush with natural preparations or sea salt.
- If your condition permits, exercise regularly as part of your daily life, including activities like scrubbing floors, cleaning windows, and so on, as well as exercise programs such as yoga, dance, sports, and martial arts.
- Avoid using electric cooking devices (ovens or ranges) or micro-wave ovens. Convert to a gas or wood stove at the earliest opportunity.
- It is best to minimize the frequent use of color television and computer display units.
- Include some large green plants in your house to freshen and enrich the oxygen content of the air in your home.

3. Dietary Adjustments for Infertility and Reproductive Disorders━━━━

So far we have looked at the *Standard Macrobiotic Diet*. To relieve obesity and eating disorders it is necessary to adjust this diet for some period of time, usually about two to three months, until the condition begins to improve.

All eating disorders reflect a basic extremism or imbalance in the body, therefore it is important in all cases to avoid overly one-sided eating. Try to present a balanced mix of ingredients and aesthetic factors such as colors, textures, and tastes in all meals. Also, it is preferable to avoid extremes of eating patterns, such as skipping one or more meals and then eating a great deal.

Proper chewing is essential for good digestion and assimilation; each mouthful can be chewed at least thirty to fifty times, or until the food is fully liquified and well-mixed with saliva. Avoid sleeping for at least three hours after eating, as this causes stagnation and weakness in the intestines.

The following are general guidelines for adjusting one's diet for obesity and eating disorders.

1. *Whole Cereal Grains:* ─────────────────────

A. *For Obesity:* Emphasize short-grain brown rice, millet, barley, pearl barley (*hato mugi*), and whole corn dishes. Buckwheat and cracked grains may be used occasionally. Minimize the intake of flour products, with the exception of occasional noodles, oats in any form, sweet brown rice, and seitan (wheat gluten).

B. *For Anorexia:* Emphasize short- and medium-grain brown rice, millet, and sweet brown rice. Whole oats may be used occasionally. Seitan and mochi may be used regularly in small amounts. Grain soups may be eaten regularly. Limit the intake of flour products and bread.

C. *For Bulimia:* Emphasize short-, medium- and long-grain brown rice, barley, and whole corn. Cracked grains may be used as well. Limit the intake of flour products and breads, oats in any form, seitan, mochi, and sweet rice.

2. Soups: ───────────────────────────

A. *For Obesity:* Limit volume to one or two bowls of soup per day. Make sure to have a small amount of sea vegetable (wakame or kombu) in your soup daily. Daikon radish and shiitake mushrooms may be used frequently in soups for help in dissolving fats.

B. *For Anorexia:* It is important to have hot or warm miso soup every day. Soups should not be overly salty and should frequently include root and sweet round vegetables, and sea vegetables. Soups containing grains, beans, or mochi may be used from time to time.

C. *For Bulimia:* Soups should be lightly seasoned with miso or tamari soy sauce. A mild sour taste can be achieved with rice or barley vinegar, umeboshi, or fresh lemon juice. Frequently include as ingredients shiitake mushrooms, leafy greens, and daikon radish.

3. Vegetables: ───────────────────────────

A. *For Obesity:* Emphasize fibrous leafy vegetables such as kale, watercress, radish or turnip greens, and sweet round or root vegetables. Lotus root (fresh or dried) and both fresh and dried daikon radish are useful in eliminating excess water and fat. Raw vegetables and salads may be eaten from time to time, along with occasional garnishes of grated raw daikon or chopped scallions. Boiled or pressed salads may be used often. A dish of sautéed vegetables may be eaten occasionally, but limit deep-frying as well as baked-vegetable dishes.

B. *For Anorexia:* Emphasize root vegetables, sweet round vegetables, and hard or fibrous leafy vegetables. *Nishime* style dishes, and stews or thicker vegetable soups may be used often. Sautéed vegetables may be used on occasion. Limit or avoid vegetables listed as "occasional use." Small amounts of pressed salad, quick pickles, or occasionally, vegetables pickled in miso or rice bran and sea salt may be eaten to enhance intestinal functioning.

C. *For Bulimia:* All vegetables listed as "regular use" and "occasional use" may be used, with an emphasis on lightly steamed, boiled, or water-sautéed vegetables. Temporarily, limit cooking with oil, and baked vegetables. Lightly pickled vegetables, and pressed and boiled salads may be eaten daily. Small amounts of raw salad may be eaten from time to time, depending on the season.

4. Beans and Bean Products: ────────────────────────

A. *For Obesity:* Moderate portions of azuki beans, chick-peas, black soybeans, and brown lentils may be emphasized. Tempeh and tofu may be used regularly, in small amounts.

B. *For Anorexia:* If difficult to digest, beans can be avoided or limited to very small quantities until intestinal functioning is improved. Azuki beans, lentils, chick-peas, and black soybeans may be eaten in small amounts, and can be well-cooked and moderately seasoned with miso, tamari soy sauce or sea salt. Natto may be used often. Tofu and tempeh may be used often, preferably cooked together with kombu and/or vegetables.

C. *For Bulimia:* Emphasize small portions of azuki, chick-peas, lentils, and black soybeans. Light bean soups and lightly cooked tofu or tempeh dishes may be eaten often, and may be mildly seasoned with a sour taste, as well as with sea salt, tamari soy sauce, or miso. Regular use of natto is recommended, if desired.

5. Sea Vegetables: ────────────────────────────

A. *For Obesity:* Sea vegetables should be eaten daily. All varieties may be used, but especially emphasize various side dishes cooked together with a small amount of kombu, such as dried or fresh daikon radish, lotus root and azuki beans. Nori may be eaten daily as a condiment, and wakame should be used frequently in miso soup.

B. *For Anorexia:* All types of sea vegetables may be used. Emphasize kombu, arame, and hijiki. A side dish of arame or hijiki cooked with root or sweet vegetables and/or tofu, dried tofu or tempeh, and lightly seasoned with tamari soy sauce and several drops of sesame oil, may be eaten three to four times per week. Kombu and wakame may be eaten daily in vegetable dishes and soups.

C. *For Bulimia:* All types are fine. Emphasize kombu, nori, arame, and wakame. A side dish of either kombu, arame, or wakame, and vegetables, seasoned with a little sour taste, sweet taste, and tamari soy sauce may be eaten three to four times per week. Nori or green nori flakes may also be used regularly as a condiment.

6. Seeds, Nuts, and Snacks:

A. *For Obesity:* To establish a regular eating pattern and smooth digestive function, it is best to minimize snacking as much as possible. Limit the use of seeds, nuts, and all oily products to occasional use.

B. *For Anorexia:* Moderate snacking is fine. Seeds and nuts may be incorporated into meals. If necessary, smaller meals may be incorporated into the daily schedule. The use of well-roasted seeds and nuts, rice cakes, popcorn, and other foods which have a drying effect on the body should be used only in moderate quantities.

C. *For Bulimia:* Limit excessive snacking, if possible. Small amounts of dried fruits, lightly toasted seeds, lightly cooked vegetables, rice balls, or sushi (without fish) may be eaten when snacks are desired.

7. Seafoods:

A. *For Obesity:* Try to minimize the intake of animal products, including seafood, if strong cravings for sweets or alcohol persist, or if there is a tendency toward compulsive eating.

B. *For Anorexia:* Seafood can be eaten when craved or needed for strength, in which case a small volume (3 to 4 ounces) of white-meat fish may be used, especially boiled, steamed, lightly broiled, or in soup.

C. *For Bulimia:* Try to limit the intake of animal products to the occasional use of white-meat fish until the tendency toward compulsive eating is reduced.

8. Desserts:

A. *For Obesity:* The desire for sweet-tasting food can be satisfied whenever possible with sweet grain, vegetable, and bean dishes. If desired, a natural dessert may be eaten occasionally, particularly those made with *kuzu* starch or agar-agar (*kanten*), and sweetened with grain-based syrups. Reduce the intake of desserts made with flour.

B. *For Anorexia:* Desserts made from sweetened grains, vegetables, or beans, and sweetened with grain syrups or amazake may be used often. Limit the intake of raw fruit. Cooked fruits, especially when cooked with kuzu, may be eaten on occasion. Eat fewer desserts prepared with flour or processed grains.

C. *For Bulimia:* Dried fruits and lightly cooked fruits may be eaten three or four times a week, particularly cooked with agar-agar or kuzu. Small amounts of raw fruits may also be used on occasion. Limit the intake of desserts prepared with flour. If craved, a small amount of citrus, such as several slices of orange, mandarin orange, or tangerine, may be eaten, especially if there has be a recent pattern of vomiting.

9. *Seasonings:*

A. *For Obesity:* Sea salt, miso, and tamari soy sauce may be used regularly, provided the food does not have a markedly salty taste. Small amounts of sesame or dark (roasted) sesame oil may be used occasionally in cooking, but raw oil is best avoided in dressings. Other macrobiotic seasonings (ginger, rice vinegar, etc.) may be used occasionally. Avoid strong spices such as garlic, pepper, or curry.

B. *For Anorexia:* Seasonings may be used to provide a slightly stronger taste, but care should be taken that the amount used does not induce excessive thirst or muscle tightness. Oil may be used more often, but in small amounts, and in cooking only. Macrobiotic-quality pungent and sweet seasonings may be used more often; sour-tasting seasonings are best limited.

C. *For Bulimia:* All seasonings may be used provided that the resulting taste is very mild. The use of oil can be limited unless fats are strongly craved, in which case a small amount of good-quality oil may be used in sautéing. Macrobiotic-quality seasonings with a sweet or sour taste may be used often; mildly pungent flavors, such as chopped scallions or grated raw daikon radish, may be used frequently. Avoid spices.

10. *Beverages:*

A. *For Obesity:* Avoid chilled or iced drinks as well as stimulating beverages such as coffee or commercial teas. Drink only when thirsty.

B. *For Anorexia:* Small amounts of hot beverages may be consumed regularly, depending on thirst. Avoid cold or chilled drinks and limit the intake of vegetable or fruit juices. Mildly bitter-tasting teas such as burdock, dandelion root, chicory, or roasted grain and bean "coffees," and Mu tea may be used on occasion.

C. *For Bulimia:* Drink only when thirsty. If cold beverages are craved, mildly cool twig tea or cereal grain teas may be drunk. If desired, a small amount of fresh vegetable or temperate-climate juice may be taken from time to time, preferably at room temperature.

11. *Condiments:*

For All Disorders: All macrobiotic table condiments may be used in moderation, taking care that they do not impart an overly salty taste to the food. Homemade gomashio, made with a proportion of 14 to 16 parts roasted sesame seeds to 1 part sea salt, may be used regularly, as well as baked and ground kombu or wakame powder, alone, or ground with crushed, toasted sesame or pumpkin seeds. Toasted nori and green nori flakes may be used regularly. Stronger condiments such as tekka, shio kombu, and the nori-tamari condiment may be used occasionally.

4. Understanding Infertility and Reproductive Disorders

It is well-known that many obese people are malnourished, most often due to improper food selection coupled with an inability to assimilate the nutrients in the foods being ingested. Compulsive eating is frequently the body's unconscious attempt to achieve a condition of stasis or balance.

All three eating disorders are characterized by a history of dietary extremes and poor assimilation, resulting generally from the poor condition of the intestinal tract, kidneys and adrenal glands, and reproductive organs, which are the primary sites of excess fat and mucus accumulation. This excess accumulation results from the over-consumption of dietary fats, particularly from eggs, dairy products, meats, flour products, and overeating in general. The condition is exacerbated by the intake of refined sugars and foods such as iced soft drinks, cold tropical-fruit juices, ice cream and other chilled dairy products, as well as raw fruits and vegetables, all of which have a chilling effect on the body.

The body normally eliminates these excesses through the eliminatory organs, the lungs, and the skin. If these organs become overburdened, the body begins to store excess under the skin and around the organs. At this point, not only is the individual unable to fully utilize the foods being eaten, but also he or she begins to lose the natural sensitivity to the external environment. This loss of sensitivity is accentuated by the increasingly common use of synthetic and artificial products.

It is not unusual to discover that many of the compulsively obese or bulimics do much of their eating in secret, frequently becoming alienated from their family and friends, and losing interest in the world around them. Such people are also often irritable and impatient. Such behavior is frequently a manifestation of an ill-functioning liver and gall bladder, both of which are prime sites of excess accumulation.

Also frequently implicated in eating disorders is *hypoglycemia* and other imbalances of the spleen and pancreas. In Oriental medicine, these imbalances are associated with feelings of depression, worry, or self-pity, coupled with a sense of being unable to control one's self and hence, one's eating. In the macrobiotic view, biology precedes psychology. Thus, the elimination of dietary excesses and partial, chemicalized, and adulterated foods leads inevitably, if gradually, to perceptible changes in one's mental and emotional condition. This occurs simultaneously with the re-establishment of physiological balance. The signs of a healthy spleen, pancreas, and intestinal tract include optimism, cheerfulness, and a compassion and sympathy extending not only to others, but to one's self as well.

The macrobiotic approach to obesity and eating disorders therefore involves a reduced intake of dietary fats, the elimination of stored excess fats and mucus, and the ingestion of a diet composed primarily of complex carbohydrates and vegetable-quality protein, which will improve overall organ functioning.

Although this book is basically concerned with dietary adjustments, it is also important to stay mentally and physically active and to maintain good relationships with the people and the world around us.

5. Menu Planning ▬▬▬▬▬▬▬▬▬

When planning a menu, there are several factors to consider.

1. The relative proportions of grains, vegetables, soup, beans, and so on in a meal as recommended in the *Standard Macrobiotic Diet.*

2. Adjustments for obesity and eating disorders (see chapter on *Dietary Adjustments for Obesity and Eating Disorders*).

3. Making sure that there is variety in your meals by varying:
   A. *The types of vegetables and grains used.* Everyday have some kind of root vegetable, fresh and leafy greens and, in some form, a small amount of sea vegetable. It is helpful to have brown rice everyday, but there are many ways to vary this basic dish as you will see in the menu examples.
   B. *The seasonings, condiments, and pickles used.* (It is preferred that one has a small amount of pickles daily.)
   C. *The cooking methods employed.* Everyday, have some quickly boiled or blanched greens, as well as pressure-cooked or longer-time cooked items.
   D. *The sizes, shapes, colors, and textures from dish to dish.* Use attractive garnishes to brighten your meals.

4. *Seasonal and climatic adjustments.* For hot weather, emphasize more fresh, lightly boiled or steamed vegetables, salads, less cooking time, and less oil and salt. For colder weather, emphasize more hearty, rich dishes, stews and thick soups, protein such as found in beans, root vegetables, and a little more salt and oil.

5. *Adjustments for the time of day.* Beans, hardy dishes, and stronger seasonings are best eaten for dinner. It is recommended that lunches and breakfasts be kept simple and light, otherwise one may feel heavy and sluggish throughout the day. Soft porridges and whole-grain cereals are delicious for breakfast.

6. *Adjustments for age.* For babies, younger children, and elderly persons, serve more soft foods and sweet-tasting vegetables with a minimum amount of seasonings. It is preferred that babies do not eat any salt at all. Teens and adults can have more seasonings and more crisp, solid vegetables.

7. *Life-style adjustments.* People doing more physical exercise, work,

and activities need more protein and hardy, rich dishes than do those who are more sedentary.

8. *Use as much of your leftovers as possible.* The menus below disregard leftovers to emphasize variety. Normally, a grain or bean dish, for example, can last for several days or more. Besides simply reheating leftovers, you can rework them into a new format; for instance, last night's dinner rice can be this morning's soft rice. Or you might want to add a few pieces of tofu when heating up yesterday's root vegetables. The possibilities are endless. All this adds more appeal and variety to your meals. It is most important, however, to have fresh, quickly boiled or blanched leafy greens everyday. Therefore, boil only as many greens as you can have in one meal.

A General Seven Day Menu Suitable for all Eating Disorders ————

	BREAKFAST	LUNCH	DINNER
1.	Celery miso soup Soft rice with wakame powder Bancha tea	Udon in broth Boiled cabbage Takuan pickle Mugicha tea	Barley soup Pressure-cooked brown rice Azuki beans/squash/kombu Arame with dried daikon Boiled mustard greens Onion pickles Bancha tea

2.	Millet porridge
	Shiso condiment
	Grated daikon with
	  nori strips
	Grain coffee
		Rice balls
		Boiled salad
		Miso pickles
		Bancha tea
			Tofu/watercress/tamari
			  broth
			Millet with squash
			Boiled cauliflower &
			  broccoli
			Kombu/carrot rolls
			Ginger pickles
			Mugicha tea

3.	Miso soup with
	  scallions
	Creamy *kasha* with
	  gomashio
	Bancha tea
		Squash soup
		Sesame seed rice
		Boiled broccoli
		Bancha tea
			Corn soup with kuzu
			Brown rice and chick-peas
			Steamed kale with tamari-
			  ginger sauce
			Sauerkraut
			Bancha tea

4. | Miso soft rice Chinese cabbage pickles | *Arepas* Boiled kale Tamari-onion pickles | Miso soup with wakame & daikon Barley and rice |
    | Mugicha tea | Bancha tea | Nishime vegetables & tempeh Boiled salad Amazake pudding Bancha tea |

5. | Barley porridge with scallions & nori Red radish pickles Bancha tea | Millet & cauliflower Boiled Chinese cabbage Miso pickles Mugicha tea | Carrot soup Rice and rye Hijiki/dried tofu/carrot/ onion Watercress sushi Quick daikon pickles Bancha tea |

6. | Scrambled tofu with corn Brown rice Grain coffee | Sushi Steamed collard greens & carrots Mugicha tea | Clear broth Boiled millet Daikon/lotus/shiitake nishime Steamed kale Cauliflower pickles Rice pudding Bancha tea |

7. | Soft millet with squash Daikon-top pickles Bancha tea | Onion miso soup Roasted rice Pressed salad Bancha tea | Celery soup Brown rice with pearl barley Arame with tempeh & onions Turnip greens with sesame/ tamari sauce Shio nori Mugicha tea |

6. Cookware ▬▬▬▬▬▬▬▬▬▬▬▬

Along with stocking the kitchen with good food, you need to equip it with a collection of essential cookware. Having the right tools in front of you makes all the difference in your cooking experience by freeing your mind to work with a more relaxed and creative attitude. This naturally has a profound effect on your well-being as well as affecting the quality, taste, and appeal of your meals. Also, some types of kitchen equipment should best be avoided as they may be detrimental to your health, while others are a must for their beneficial influences. Listed below is a checklist of what you will need.

1. We recommend a gas stove as opposed to an electric one. There are several reasons for this:

    A. Electricity dissipates the molecular structure and strength of food by causing the electrons to bounce out of the atomic field, leaving the atom very unstable. Gas, on the other hand, just bounces the molecules around, while leaving them intact.

    B. It is very hard to fine-tune your cooking with electricity. It is a conductive heat which first warms the coils and then the pot and its contents from the bottom up. You can not change the temperature quickly when turning to high or low because it takes some time to cool or heat the pot. It is difficult to cook uniformly, and it is possible that ingredients at the bottom of the pan can burn while those at the top need more cooking. A gas flame heats the surrounding air. The food is cooked much more evenly and the temperature can be adjusted immediately (a pot of water will instantly stop boiling the moment you turn off the flame, for example). Meals are more well cooked.

    C. Because of these drawbacks in electric cooking, a person may not feel satisfied with the meal and may crave strong salt or animal food (to counter the yin and weakening effects) which in turn causes a craving for excessive sweets and other yin foods. In other words, it becomes more of a struggle to eat in a balanced manner and thus to stay on the macrobiotic diet.

A microwave oven is definitely out of the picture and should be avoided, particularly if someone in the family is sick. It zaps food with radioactive waves at three-billion cycles per second (a regular electric stove runs at 60-cycles per second and is actually a low form of radiation). It disintegrates instead of cooks and can cause the same effect in our body. Not only is it not a help in regaining health, but it is suspected to contribute to certain types of illnesses. Recent studies have shown that foods prepared with a microwave oven produce tumors in mice.

After gas, wood is the best source of heat (followed by coal or charcoal) though it is impractical for most modern homes. It has a peaceful energy and at the same time it gives great strength to our foods.

2. Several stainless-steel pots of varying sizes. The steel does not interfere with the energies of the food. It is best to avoid aluminum because it is a poisonous substance and under high temperatures or when cooking very acidic (sweet) or alkaline (salty) foods, harmful toxins are released and mixed in with your ingredients.

    Cookware made out of glass (like Pyrex), earthenware, and enamelware are also excellent materials to cook in. (Be careful that you do not pour cold water into a heated enamel pot or leave it empty over a flame as this will cause it to crack. Let it cool off before washing it. It is also easily scratched so do not clean it with a steel-wool scrubber and use a wooden spoon when handling food inside it.)

3. At least one pressure cooker (stainless or enamel steel). This is an ideal pot for cooking grains, beans, root vegetables (like big chunks of burdock), squash, or anything that takes a long time to soften. The nutrients are better retained and everything is cooked more thoroughly, quickly, and with more energy than when prepared in a regular pot.

    To use, put ingredients inside (not more than ¾ full), cover (don't forget to put the weight attachment on top), and over a medium-high flame, bring to pressure. You can tell the pressure is up when there is a lot of hissing and the weight begins to jiggle and shake. Then, immediately turn down the flame and, if needed, place a heat deflector underneath. Simmer (anywhere from 5 to 10 minutes to an hour or more depending on what is inside) until the food is done. Take the pot off the stove and let the pressure come down. You can let it come down naturally or rinse the pot under cold running water in the sink. This brings it down right away.

Before you cook, carefully take a good look at the cover. Inspect the hole (on which you place the weight) and make sure that it is not clogged. Otherwise, an explosion can occur when the pressure is high. Also, look at the rubber rings on the inside of the lid and in the pot itself where the rings touch. Remove any bits of food or other substances which may be stuck there as they will create a gap where steam can escape and as a result, the pressure will never build up.

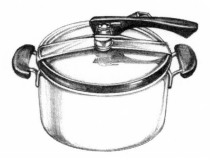

Fig. 9   Pressure Cooker

4. Several cast-iron skillets for roasting and sautéing. Season them when you first get them and from time to time thereafter. To do this, wash and dry them thoroughly. Rub sesame oil all over (outside also) with a paper towel. You can coat the inside by rotating and tilting the pan over a flame. Place them in the oven at 225° to 250°F. for 2 to 3 hours. Then, let them sit for a few hours until they cool. Seasoning prevents the pans from rusting. For the same reason, do not soak them in hot, soapy water, and dry them thoroughly over a low flame after you wash them.

5. One deep cast-iron pot for deep-frying. Cast iron is the best material to hold the intense heat of the oil.

6. Baking containers including pie plates, bread pans, muffin tins and so on. Again, avoid aluminum.

7. An optional *wok* (a Chinese-style skillet). The cast-iron skillets can effectively cover your sautéing needs but a wok is great for quick, light and fast cooking vegetables and fish.

8. Several stainless-steel mixing bowls in different sizes for washing and mixing your food.

9. Large wooden serving bowls for your grains. Wood allows grains to breathe and retards their spoilage as it absorbs any excess water. You need to oil the bowls periodically to prevent them from cracking. Heat some sesame oil, pour it into a completely dry bowl which you rotate until the inside is thoroughly oiled. Oil the outside also, with a brush or paper towel. Let it sit for a few hours until it dries completely.

10. Various other attractive serving containers made of glass, china, or ceramics. (Plastic is to be avoided.)

11. A stainless-steel or bamboo steamer.

12. A colander for rinsing noodles and other foods.

13. A fine-mesh strainer for washing seeds and grains.

14. A *suribachi* and pestle for making gomashio and other condiments. This is a Japanese ceramic bowl with grooves, made for crushing roasted sesame seeds, sea vegetables and so on.

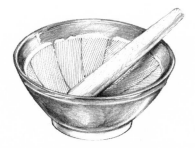

Fig. 10   Suribachi and Pestle

15. A food mill for pureeing cooked grains and vegetables. (An electric blender is more disruptive to the energies of foods. Instead of using one on a regular basis, save it for parties or special occasions when working with large volumes.)

16. A grain mill for grinding grains and nuts into flour. Flour is best when used soon after grinding. It immediately starts to oxidize and begins to lose some of its nutrients. Also, it is most delicious when fresh. (Your local natural food store may have a good supply of flour as well.)

17. A pickle press for making pickles and pressed salads.

18. An earthenware crock with a wide mouth is good for making bran pickles, among other things.

19. Tea pot or kettle. Avoid aluminum.

20. A tea strainer for straining out leaves and twigs when serving the tea. A bamboo strainer, found in natural food and Oriental stores, is the best one to use.

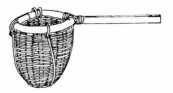

Fig. 11   Tea Strainer

21. Large glass jars for storing grains, beans, nuts, seeds, and other foods, as well as for making pickles.

22. Wooden cutting boards. Keep a separate one for fish and animal foods as their bacteria can have a toxic effect on vegetables.

23. Knives. The square-shaped Oriental knives are the easiest and the most efficient. They come in:
    A. carbon (which has a good sharp edge but rusts and chips easily),
    B. stainless steel (which does not rust but is not as sharp), and
    C. high-grade carbon with stainless steel which does not rust and is sharp as well (but is more expensive).

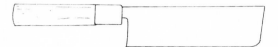

Fig. 12   Vegetable Knife

To protect the carbon knives, wash them in warm, soapy water and dry them immediately, as soon as you use them. If rust starts to appear, scrape it off with a steel-wool scrubber. Along with keeping your knives as dry as possible, they may be coated with a little sesame oil after use.

You will want to get a sharpening stone to keep the edges of knifes sharp. Oil the stone with a vegetable oil or rinse it in water before you use it. Tilt the knife at a twenty-degree angle and sweep the blade against the stone in several circular motions. Use one hand to press down upon the blade while the other hand holds the knife and moves it in circles. Sharpen the entire length of the edge. You may choose to sharpen just one side for more control (the right side for right handers and the left side for lefties). Do not use this knife for bread as its blade may be destroyed.

24. A bread knife. The best knife for cutting bread has a long, thin blade with a serrated edge.

25. A grater, most often used in macrobiotic cooking for grating fresh ginger, daikon, carrots, onions, lotus root, jinenjo, and taro potato.

26. A vegetable peeler, good for removing skins of cucumbers, apples and so on, when necessary.

27. A flame or heat deflector. This thin metal plate is placed underneath the pot or pressure cooker to even the flame and to help prevent the food from burning. Do not use the white asbestos deflectors as asbestos is poisonous.

28. An oil skimmer for lifting small bits of batter and food from tempura oil as well as for lifting vegetables from a pot of water.

29. A natural-bristle brush for brushing oil into skillets, cookie sheets, muffin tins, pie plates, and so on. Any small, clean, unused brush can be used.

30. Drop tops. These tops fit inside the pot and sit right on top of the food you are cooking, especially effective in cooking beans. They add some pressure but let steam escape and thus the food is cooked more thoroughly and softens more quickly.

31. Drop tops for pickles made in a keg such as bran pickles. A wooden one is best. A heavy stone or weight is placed on top for pressure. A plate is a good substitute if a wooden top cannot be found.

32. A vegetable brush with natural bristles is best for washing vegetables. They can be found in natural or Oriental food stores.

33. Wooden spoons for stirring, mixing, scooping and serving food before and after you cook. Wood has the best energy in interaction with your food and is more gentle to your pots, pans and bowls. Wooden spoons do not scratch cookware.

34. A bamboo rice paddle for handling and serving your grains.

35. Soup ladles.

36. Rubber spatula for scraping batter, puréed food and so on from clean bowls.

37. A metal spatula for turning food over.

38. Cooking chopsticks. These are longer than the table version.

39. A rolling pin.

40. Measuring cups and spoons.

41. Sushi mats for making sushi and for covering cooked food. (They let air circulate and help retard spoilage.)

42. Bamboo mats. Also for covering food.

43. One hundred percent cotton cheesecloths, used as a cover when making pickles and also for making little sacks to contain foods in cooking (sort of like a tea bag).

44. Paper towels.

7. Cooking Attitude ▬▬▬▬▬▬▬

Besides having good-quality food and proper cookware, to be a good cook, the right attitude and frame of mind are also necessary. Here is another check list.

1. Leave all your worries, problems, and angers behind as you relax your mind and body into a peaceful, calm state of being. All your thoughts and emotions get mixed into the food and have an effect on anyone who eats it. Here are some things, among others, which you can think about as you cook:

   A. Pour your love and healing vibrations into your food and imagine that whoever eats it will become healthier and happier.

   B. Imagine that the food has the power to help realize everyone's dreams and that with this tool you have the ability to vitalize and inspire whole civilizations, because you do.

   C. In your mind, thank the farmer, trucker, store keeper, nature, the food itself, cookware companies, and anyone else who has made it possible for you to have these wonderful ingredients and utensiles in front of you.

   D. Imagine that you are composing a symphony or painting a masterpiece as you combine colors, textures, tastes, and smells into beautiful and dynamic combinations. Release your creativity and intuition more and more, day by day.

   E. Realize that there is always more to learn. Do not ever become arrogant and think that you know it all. Be open and you can learn from everyone around you. We all have different perspectives and ideas and therefore we all have something to offer.

2. Clean and organize your kitchen and surroundings before, during, and after you cook.

3. If you have long hair, tie it back to help prevent it from catching on fire, as well as from falling into the food. Wear a clean apron and roll up your sleeves.

4. Work quickly, calmly, and efficiently, economically making the most of your time. Avoid munching while you cook as this will really slow you down.

5. Keep other activities and distractions to a minimum and concentrate all your energies in your cooking.

6. When making your menu, first look at all your leftovers and older vegetables and use these first. Do not waste any food. Avoid buying more perishables than you need. Look first at your supply before you go shopping.

7. Develop your intuition and common sense so that you can appropriately adapt your meals to the weather, the season, the people for whom you are cooking, with their daily needs and changes, your own moods, and any other influencing factors for that particular place and time.

8. Keep your meals simple. Do not mash together a lot of different ingredients into one dish. Go light on your seasonings and use them mainly to draw out and enhance the natural flavors of your food.

9. Decorate your food beautifully, set the table using appealing tableware, and make your dining area comfortable and aesthetically pleasing. This enhances your appetite and dining experience.

10. Take the time and place to relax, sit down, and peacefully enjoy your meal with appreciation. Chew your food thoroughly, the saliva helps digestion. Also, it is best not to eat unless one is truly hungry.

8. Grains and Grain Products ━━━

Grains: ━━━━━━━━━━━━━━━━━━━━━━━━

The most helpful dishes for regular use include:

For All Disorders:

Short-grain brown rice, pressure-cooked
Azuki beans and rice
Millet; rice and millet; millet and sweet vegetables

For Obesity:

Barley soup; rice and barley
Pearl barley (hato mugi)

For Anorexia:

Sweet brown rice and rice
Seitan stew, seitan with vegetables
Grain soups

For Bulimia:

Barley soup; rice and barley
Whole corn dishes

Grains stored in a cool, dark, dry location can be kept indefinitely. Use organically grown grains whenever possible. To retain the maximum energy of your grains, leave them unhusked until just before you cook with them, if possible.

Before you wash grains, spread a handful at a time onto a plate and remove any stones and other debris which may be mixed in. Then, place the grains in a bowl (the lightweight stainless-steel mixing bowls are excellent for this), cover with cold water, and very gently stir and rinse off any dirt that floats to the top. Repeat until the water becomes clear. Then, place the grain in a colander or strainer. Wash quickly to help retain as many nutrients in the grain as possible.

There are several kinds of grains that are available:

Brown Rice:

Brown rice, being the easiest to digest, is the most suitable grain for daily use. You can have it everyday, regardless of whether you are in the transitional, healing, or standard phase. We eat it at almost every meal. The other grains serve as variations, either as a substitute or as an additional ingredient in a meal. We mainly use four types of rice:

1. *Short grain:* This is the variety with the hardiest taste and energy, and the most effective one for creating a healthy, balanced condition in our body. Use this one most of the time, especially in the winter.

2. *Medium grain:* This is more soft and moist and is a nice variation.

3. *Long grain:* This is light and fluffy, excellent for fried rice, and makes a great alternative in the summer and in warmer climates.

4. *Sweet rice:* This is even more sweet and glutinous than the short grain and is quite sticky. Sweet rice can be added to other grains periodically for a sweeter taste, and also serves as a base for *ohagi*, mochi and amazake.

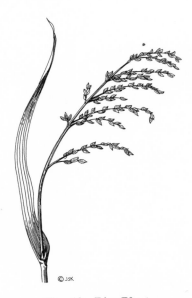

Fig. 13   Rice Plant

We recommend pressure-cooking your rice most of the time. This form of preparation cooks the grains more thoroughly, making them easier to digest. Pressure-cooked grains are less soggy, and are sweeter and more healing. Along with the help of a pressure cooker there are two ways to make your grain softer, sweeter, and more digestible:

1. *Non-soaking:* Start cooking the grain very slowly over a low flame, in an uncovered pressure cooker. Do not put any salt in yet so that it will take more time to come to a boil. When it comes to a boil, add the salt, cover, and bring up to pressure (it is up when the gauge hisses). Then, place a heat deflector underneath (make sure the flame is on medium-low) and simmer for 45 to 50 minutes.

2. *Soaking:* Soak the rice (covered with cold water) for 3 to 5 hours or overnight. Place in the pressure cooker (along with the soaking water). This time, add salt and cover right away (otherwise it may turn out too soggy). Put on a medium-high flame and bring up to pressure. When it is up, turn the flame down to medium-low, place a heat deflector underneath, and simmer for 45 to 50 minutes.

Basic Brown Rice (Pressure-Cooked)
(Use everyday, the principal food for all conditions.)

3 cups brown rice
3¾–4½ cups spring water
3 pinches sea salt

Pressure-cook following one of the above methods. Let the pressure come down completely before removing the cover. Scoop out the rice, with a wet rice paddle or wooden spoon, into a wooden bowl as you separate and air out the lumps.

The bottom rice can be mixed in if it is not burnt. Keep the brown side turned down and totally covered to help keep it soft. If the bottom is really stuck to the pot, keep a 1-inch layer of rice in the pot, put the lid back on, and let it sit for 20 to 30 minutes. The warmth of the fresh rice will help to loosen and soften the bottom.

Keep the rice covered with a bamboo or sushi mat. Either of these mats will protect the rice while letting it have air to breathe. Then dish the rice into individual bowls and serve. Serves 6.

There are many variations that you can use. Below are four helpful recipes followed by a partial listing of other variations.

Azuki Bean Rice
(Helps strengthen the kidneys and adrenals.)

2½ cups brown rice
½ cup azuki beans
4½ cups spring water
3 pinches sea salt
1 strip kombu, 3″–6″

Wash azuki beans and boil them with the kombu in 2 cups of water for 10 to 15 minutes, until the water becomes red. Cool the beans till they are lukewarm. Wash the rice, put it in the pressure cooker with the beans and the red, boiled juice. Use pressure-cooking method #1 (*Non-soaking*) and follow the directions for *Basic Brown Rice*. Or you can soak the rice and beans together overnight and use method #2 (*Soaking*). Serves 6.

Lotus Seed Rice
(The addition of lotus seeds makes this dish especially strengthening for the lungs and the kidneys.)

2½ cups rice
½ cup lotus seeds
4½ cups spring water
3 pinches sea salt

Wash and soak lotus seeds and rice 3 to 4 hours or overnight. Pressure-cook using method #2 and following the directions for *Basic Brown Rice* (*Pressure-cooked*). Serves 6.

Sesame Seed Rice
(Helps improve general vitality.)

2½ cups brown rice
½ cup roasted white or black sesame seeds
3¾–4½ cups spring water
3 pinches sea salt

Wash and quickly roast white or black sesame seeds (being careful not to burn them) in a skillet, stirring with a wooden spoon, until a nutty fragrance is emitted. Combine with all the other ingredients and cook as in *Basic Brown Rice* (*Pressure-cooked*). Serves 6.

Sweet Rice and Millet
(Strengthens spleen, pancreas, and stomach.)

2 cups sweet rice
1 cup millet
4 cups spring water
3 pinches sea salt

Wash and combine all the ingredients and cook as in *Basic Brown Rice* (*Pressure-cooked*), method #2 (minus the soaking) for 40 to 45 minutes. Serves 6.
Other variations include:

1) $2\frac{1}{2}$ cups rice + $\frac{1}{2}$ cup barley ($4\frac{1}{2}$ cups water)
2) 2 cups rice + 1 cup millet ($4\frac{1}{2}$ cups water)
3) 2 cups rice + 1 cup sweet rice
4) $2\frac{1}{2}$ cups rice + $\frac{1}{2}$ cup wheat berries (soaked overnight)
5) $2\frac{1}{2}$ cups rice + $\frac{1}{2}$ cup roasted sunflower seeds
6) $2\frac{1}{2}$ cups rice + $\frac{1}{2}$ cup chick-peas (soaked overnight)
7) 2 cups rice + 1 cup dried chestnuts
8) 2 cups rice + 1 cup fresh corn kernels (3 cups water)
9) $2\frac{1}{2}$ cups rice + $\frac{1}{2}$ cup wild rice
10) $2\frac{1}{2}$ cups rice + $\frac{1}{2}$ cup roasted walnuts
11) 2 cups rice + 1 umeboshi plum (instead of salt)
12) Bancha tea instead of water
13) $2\frac{1}{2}$ cups rice + 1 cup squash
14) $2\frac{1}{2}$ cups rice + $\frac{1}{2}$ cup roasted black or yellow soybeans

You can also boil the rice once in a while. Boiling does not give the strength of pressure-cooking but it is a great alternative when you want something lighter, more yin, and to add some variety. When eating boiled rice, make sure to chew well. You can dry-roast the rice before boiling it for variation.

Basic Brown Rice (Boiled)

2 cups brown rice, washed
4 cups spring water
2 pinches sea salt

Put washed rice into a pot (preferably with a heavy lid) with water and salt. Bring to a boil, then lower the flame, place a heat deflector underneath, and simmer for about 1 hour or until all the water has been absorbed. Wet a wooden spoon or rice paddle (so the rice will not stick to it) and dish out the rice into a wooden bowl. Cover with a sushi or bamboo mat.
(*Option:* You can roast the rice in a skillet till golden brown before boiling it. This gives more flavor. Gently stir the grains

in the skillet with a wooden spoon to prevent them from
burning.) Serves 4.

When someone is not feeling well, we often make soft rice. It is
more soothing and is easier on the digestive system. A bowl of it is
usually accompanied by an umeboshi plum which also helps digestion.
Even if you are feeling fine, this makes a delicious porridge. If you
leave out the salt, this also makes a perfect food for babies and young
children.

Soft Rice (Plain)
(A good healing dish.)

> 1 cup brown rice
> 5 cups water
> 1 pinch sea salt

Cook as in *Basic Brown Rice* (*Pressure-cooked*). You can also
boil it by simmering it overnight over a low flame and a heat
deflector. If you do so, use 10 cups of water to every cup of
rice. Serves 5.

People suffering from weak digestion could use a bowl of miso
soup or a bowl of soft miso rice regularly. Below is a soft-rice recipe
made from cooked brown rice.

Ojiya (Soft Rice with Miso)
(Have often while healing.)

> 2 cups leftover cooked brown rice
> 4–5 cups spring water
> 3 Tbsps. (or to taste) miso instead of salt
> 1 strip kombu, 4″–6″
> 3–4 sliced scallions

Wash, soak, and slice the kombu and place it in the bottom of
a pot or pressure cooker. Add the rice and water and bring
them to a boil or to pressure. Turn the flame to low, place
a deflector underneath, and simmer or pressure-cook for
½ hour. Add 1 tablespoon or so of water to the miso and stir
it in until the miso becomes a puree. Uncover the rice (wait
until the pressure is gone if using a pressure cooker) and then
put it back onto the stove. Mix in the miso, simmer for another

3 to 5 minutes, and turn off the flame. Garnish with sliced scallions and serve immediately. Serves 4 to 5.

Rice Cream with Nori and Umeboshi
(Rice cream is a dish with special healing qualities. It helps purify blood and lymph.)

1 cup dry-roasted brown rice
3–6 cups spring water
1 pinch sea salt
1 sheet toasted nori
1 umeboshi plum
Cheesecloth

Pressure-cook with salt and water for 1 hour following directions for *Basic Brown Rice* (*Pressure-cooked*). Make a sack out of clean cheesecloth. Cool off the cooked rice, place some inside the sack and squeeze out as much of the creamy liquid as you can. Reheat and serve with nori and an umeboshi plum. The leftover pulp can be eaten separately or added to soup or vegetable dishes. (Occasionally, instead of soaking the rice in the beginning, you can dry-roast it in a skillet until golden brown.) Serves 2.

Musubi (Rice Ball)
(Great for lunches, picnics, and trips, it is also a very strengthening, stabilizing way to eat rice.)

1 cup cooked short-grain (sticks well) brown rice
2 quarter sheets nori (a sheet cut in half and then half again)
1 pinch sea salt
1 umeboshi plum (or ½ if it is large)

Toast nori by passing it over an open flame a few times until it becomes green but not so much that it becomes crisp and crinkly. Tear it into 4 pieces.

Wet hands (to prevent the rice from sticking to them) in a bowl of salted water, put the rice in your palms and stick an umeboshi plum in the middle (the pit may be removed if desired). Tightly mold the rice around the plum in an English-muffin shape or a flat triangle, and put it on a plate.

Wash and dry your hands. Then use a quarter of a sheet of nori on each side of the rice ball and cover with the shiny side (of the nori) on the outside. Firmly mold it on. You can then eat the rice ball or pack it up and take it on a trip to consume later. Serves 1.

Frying is a delicious way to use up leftover rice. Remember, however, that for some conditions it is recommended to limit the use of oil.

Fried Rice

> 3 cups cooked brown rice
> 1 onion, diced
> 1 sheet toasted nori
> 5 sliced scallions
> 1 Tbsp. dark sesame oil
> Tamari soy sauce to taste
> 1 tsp. grated ginger

Heat the oil in a skillet and add diced onions (drop one piece in first and if it sizzles, the oil is hot enough). Stir them a bit with a wooden spoon and then add the rice. Thoroughly mix and stir, breaking up all the big lumps of rice. You can cover, turn the flame to low, and let it heat up for about 10 minutes. Then, add soy sauce to taste and simmer for another 3 to 5 minutes or so. Break up the toasted nori into little pieces and mix into the rice, along with the scallions and ginger, at the end. Serves 2 to 3.

Mochi is a traditional Japanese dish which is eaten on festive occasions. Mochi cakes or squares are made out of pounded sweet rice. Several pieces in miso soup can help strengthen the intestines.

Mochi (Homemade)

> 4 cups sweet rice
> 4 cups water
> 4 pinches sea salt
> A handful of any finely ground flour (pastry, sweet rice,
>   arrowroot, etc.)

Cook as in *Basic Brown Rice* (*Pressure-cooked*). When done, in a wooden bowl, vigorously pound the rice with a large wooden pestle (which you wet initially and then from time to time to prevent the rice from sticking to it) until all the grains are crushed and form a smooth, sticky mass. This may take a half hour. Sprinkle some flour onto a baking sheet and layer the rice on top (up to 1-inch thick). Dry this for 1 to 2 days and then store it in the refrigerator.

When you want to have some, cut the mochi into small pieces and toast them in a skillet, with or without oil, until they become soft. This only takes a few minutes. (Turn them over when they are half done so that both sides toast evenly.) Serve them with some raw grated daikon with a few drops of tamari soy sauce added. The daikon helps in the digestion of the mochi. Serves 5 to 6.

Fortunately, you can get previously pounded brown rice mochi in some natural food stores. All you have to do is to toast it for a few minutes.

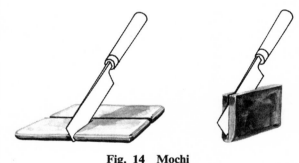

Fig. 14   Mochi

Millet:

Millet is a more yang grain, being small, round, and more alkaline. It is good for the spleen and pancreas, it helps to settle an acidic stomach, and it gives warmth. For helping to relieve blood glucose disorders, it can be considered as a major grain after rice.

It cooks fairly quickly and comes out very soft so you can, but do not need to, pressure-cook it. It can be made either light and fluffy or moist and creamy like a porridge. The fluffy style can be a little too dry, so it can often be eaten with a sauce or cooked with other ingredients. A standard combination uses squash (delicious). Other common companions are vegetables like carrots and onions as well as roasted seeds.

Millet (Dry)

1 cup millet
2 cups water
1 pinch sea salt

Wash the millet. As an option, you may roast it with or without
a tablespoon of oil in a skillet until a delicious nutty aroma is
emitted. (For those who must limit their oil intake, dry-roast
until your condition improves. Stir quickly with a wooden
spoon to prevent burning.) Bring the salt and water to a boil
and slowly and carefully add the millet. Let this come up to
a boil again. Then, cover the pot, turn the flame to medium-
low, place a heat deflector underneath, and simmer for about
30 minutes. Serves 2.

Millet Porridge

1 cup millet
4 cups boiling water
2 pinches sea salt

Bring salt and water to a boil. Wash the millet and carefully
pour it into the pot of boiling water. Bring to a boil again,
turn the flame to low, place a heat deflector underneath, cover,
and simmer for 30 minutes. Serves 3.

Millet and Squash

1 cup millet
½ cup buttercup or Hokkaido squash
2½ cups water
3 pinches sea salt

Wash and cut the squash into cubes. Remove the seeds and
trim away the brown crusted substances on the surface of the
skin, if there are any. If the skin happens to be extremely hard
(as is sometimes the case with the Hokkaido), you can slice it
off. Place the squash in a pot, put the millet on top, add water
and salt, cover, and bring to a boil. Then turn the flame to low,
place a heat deflector underneath, and simmer for 30 minutes.
Serves 2 to 3.

Other variations:

1) Millet + cauliflower (3½ cups water)
2) Millet + squash + onions, pressure-cooked 15 minutes

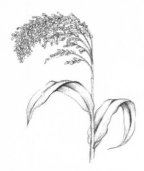

Fig. 15 Millet Plant

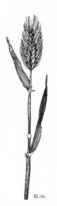

Fig. 16 Barley Plant

Barley:

Barley is usually used in combination with other grains (such as rice) and vegetables. It is very mild tasting and lends itself easily to this. Cook it just like rice. Barley is light and has a cooling, calming energy. It helps to discharge accumulated animal fats from the body.

Barley Porridge

> 1 cup barley
> 4–5 cups spring water
> 1 pinch sea salt
> Several parsley sprigs

Boil as in *Basic Brown Rice* (*Boiled*). Simmer for 1¼ to 1½ hours or until soft. Garnish with the parsley. Serves 5.

Buckwheat:

Buckwheat can grow in a very cold climate and has a short growing season. This grain gives strength, generates heat, and is good for the lungs, kidneys, and bladder. It is a great winter food. However, people with an overly tight condition should use this grain only occasionally until their condition clears up.

Buckwheat can be cooked like millet as it also cooks quickly and is a soft grain. Below is a recipe for creamy *kasha* (buckwheat).

Creamy Kasha

> 1 cup buckwheat groats
> 2 scallions
> 5 cups spring water
> 1 pinch sea salt

Wash the buckwheat and put it into a pot. Add cold water and sea salt and bring to a boil. Then turn the flame down to low, place a flame deflector underneath, and cook for 20 to 30 minutes. Wash and slice the scallions for a garnish. Serves 3.

Oats:

Oats have more protein and fat than other grains. Therefore, while they are helpful to produce more warmth in the body, they should not be taken on a daily basis as they can cause a buildup of mucus. Use about two times a week maximum during the initial healing stage, and use whole oats whenever possible.

Whole Oats

1 cup whole oats
5 cups spring water
1 pinch sea salt
1 strip kombu, 3"–6"

Wash and soak oats for 3 hours or overnight. Add kombu (it helps to cut the fat in the oats) and pressure-cook 2 hours, or boil just like brown rice. If boiling, slowly simmer over a low flame for three or more hours or overnight. Small cubes of winter squash can also be cooked along with the oats for a sweet flavor. Serves 3.

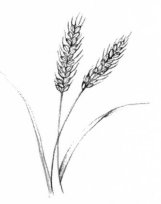

Fig. 17   Wheat Plant

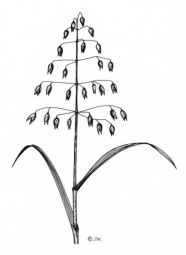

Fig. 18   Oat Plant

Wheat: ─────────────────────────────────

Wheat berries are harder to digest than other grains. They should always be soaked beforehand. Make sure you chew really well in order to insure good digestion.

Pressure-cook like rice except that the wheat berries need to be soaked for several hours or overnight. You may also need to cook them an extra 10 to 15 minutes. Use twice as much water as grain.

Wheat also comes in the form of bulghur, which has been partially boiled, dried, and then ground; and couscous, which has been refined and cracked. Both of these wheat products are convenient, as they cook very quickly, especially couscous. However, they should not be used as staple foods since a great deal of nutrition is lost in their processing. Use them as an occasional treat and for variety.

Azuki Bean Wheat Berries

2 cups wheat berries
$\frac{1}{2}$–$\frac{3}{4}$ cup azuki beans
4–5 cups spring water
2 pinches sea salt

Wash and soak wheat berries and beans together for 3 to 5 hours or overnight. Pressure-cook as in *Basic Brown Rice.* Simmer for 60 to 70 minutes. Serves 6 to 8.

Bulghur and Vegetables

1 cup bulghur
$\frac{1}{4}$ cup each diced onions, carrots, and celery
2–2$\frac{1}{4}$ cups spring water
1 pinch sea salt

Bring salt and water to a boil. Meanwhile, wash and dice the vegetables and layer them (onions on the bottom, then celery, and finally carrots on top) in another pot. Add some water (just enough to cover the vegetables) and simmer until they are soft. Then, add the bulghur, pour the boiling water on top, cover, and bring to a boil again. Turn the flame to low and simmer for 20 minutes. Serves 3.

Boiled Couscous

1 cup couscous
2$\frac{1}{2}$ cups spring water
1 pinch sea salt
Optional: 1 tsp. sesame oil

Bring the water, salt, and optional oil to a boil. Pour in the couscous, turn the flame to low, cover, and simmer for 5 minutes. Add some garnish or sauce. Serves 2.

Corn:

The corn eaten by the native American Indians was much hardier, stronger, smaller, and nutritious than most of the commercial corn available today. This grain was more effective in maintaining one's health, particularly strengthening the heart and blood vessels.

During the healing stage use only corn dishes that have been cooked whole at the beginning, such as whole corn dishes and traditional *masa*, *tortillas*, and so on. Avoid dishes that have been ground previous to any cooking, as they may cause a buildup of mucus.

There are five main types of corn available today:
1. *Sweet corn*—The regular corn on the cob.
2. *Dent corn*—Corn with dented kernels used for making cornmeal.
3. *Flour corn*—Starchy variety used in Latin American cooking.
4. *Flint corn*—Starchy variety used in Latin America Cooking.
5. *Popcorn.*

Corn on the Cob (Boiled)

Desired number of ears of fresh corn
A pot of water
Several pinches sea salt
1 Tbsp. umeboshi paste

Trim away the Corn's dry, outer leaves, but keep the fresher inner wrapping intact. Chop off the excess straggly husk ends and silk hairs on the top end of the corn. Put sea salt in the water and bring to a boil. Drop the corn in and boil for about 10 minutes. Take out the corn and serve. After unhusking you can rub on umeboshi paste (as you would with butter) if you want. Strain any leftover silk hairs from the liquid with an oil skimmer, and use this liquid for soup stock.

Dried Whole Corn (Dent, Flint, or Flour)

2 cups whole, dried corn
8 cups spring water
2 pinches sea salt
1 cup sifted wood ash

Wash and soak the corn overnight. Put the corn, 4 cups of

water, and the wood ash (no salt) in a pressure cooker. Cook
for 30 to 45 minutes. When the corn is done, put it into
a colander or strainer. Rinse out all the ash and remove the
corn skins. (If the skins are not loose enough, cook again with
more ashes for another 10 minutes.) Pressure-cook the unhulled
corn for 1 hour in a clean pot with salt and 4 more cups of
water. You can serve the corn as it is, or use it as a base for
other corn recipes. Serves 4 to 6.

Masa (Corn Dough)

   4 cups whole, dried flint or flour corn
   8–10 cups water initially and 8 more cups later
   1 cup sifted wood ash
   3–4 pinches sea salt

Follow the directions in *Dried Whole Corn* except that you use
8 to 10 cups of water in the beginning and 8 more cups after
the corn is hulled. Take out and cool the corn. Grind it in
a hand grinder (not a blender). Knead this for about 15 minutes. You can moisten it with a little water if it is too dry. If
you do not use the dough immediately, store it in the refrigerator (up to a week). This is the base for many corn recipes
such as *arepas*, tortillas, cereals, an so on.

Arepas

   3 cups masa corn dough (see above recipe)
   Boiling water
   Water to help shape the dough
   2–3 pinches sea salt
   1 Tbsp. sesame oil
   Optional: **½ cup roasted sesame seeds**

Knead the dough while mixing in salt and optional sesame
seeds. It should feel like bread dough. If it is too dry, add
a little water, and if too wet, add more dough or let it sit and
dry for a few minutes. Separate it into balls which you mold
into English-muffin shapes, except a little flatter. Boil some
water, put the balls in, and remove them when they rise to the
top.
   Heat some oil in a skillet, place the arepas inside, cover, and
cook them over a low flame for about 15 to 20 minutes. (Turn
them over halfway through to cook the other side.) If you
want, you can then slit them open and stuff them with beans
and/or vegetables. Serves 4 to 6.

Grain Products: ━━━━━━━━━━━━━━━━━━━━━━━━━━━━━━━━━━

During the initial several months, it is better to avoid flour or refined-grain products altogether. This is particularly so for any dry, roasted, or baked items such as bread, crackers, granola, and others. However, boiled whole grain flour products may be used occasionally for variety, including noodles (but avoiding buckwheat), fu, and seitan.

Remember, that for some conditions it is best to limit the consumption of bread and other grain products.

1. Noodles are a great snack and cook up very quickly. There are several types which are now available in most natural food stores.

    A. *Soba*—Long, thin, Oriental buckwheat noodles.
        1) Buckwheat with/without wheat in varying amounts
        2) Jinenjo soba (contains jinenjo flour)
        3) *Ito* soba—extra thin and light
        4) *Ramen*—Instant noodles

    B. *Udon*—Long, Oriental wholewheat noodles.
        1) Thicker than soba and contains wholewheat and sometimes unbleached, sifted white flour
        2) *Somen*—Very thin wheat noodles
        3) Ramen—Instant noodles

    C. *Pasta*—Wheat alone or in combination with other grain flours.
        1) Spaghetti
        2) Shells
        3) Spirals
        4) Elbows
        5) Ribbons
        6) Ziti
        7) Rigatoni
        8) Linguini
        9) Lasagna
        10) Alphabets, etc.

Buy these noodles, especially the ramen and pasta, from natural food stores. The ramen bought in Oriental shops may contain animal fats, sugar, MSG, chemicals, additives, and food coloring. Pasta bought in a regular store usually contain eggs which are best avoided.

To cook noodles, place them in a large pot of boiling water. (Too little water causes them to clump together.) As you put them in, stir and separate the noodles with a long chopstick to prevent them from lying side by side in a parallel fashion, otherwise they will stick together. (This precaution is basically for long thin noodles such as udon and soba.)

You can keep the flame high and add a little cold water each time the pot comes to a boil until the noodles are soft (usually about 3 times). Or you can turn the flame down a bit after adding the noodles and simmer until they are cooked. The first method is preferred as the noodles come out more firm and crisp. When done, the inside is the same color as the outside. Drain them in a colander and immediately run cold water over them. This helps to keep them from clumping together.

Avoid making them too soggy, especially if you are later going to reheat or fry them. Pay special attention to the somen and Ito soba as they cook up very quickly and are absolutely horrible when soft and mushy.

Add a pinch of salt when boiling pasta. (Udon and soba already contain salt so they do not need it.) The leftover noodle water can be used in soup stocks.

After ramen is boiled, it is generally left in the pot and the accompanying packet of dry-soup ingredients is mixed in. Read what the packet contains to make sure that the contents are healthy.

Noodles in Broth

1 pack udon or soba noodles previously boiled
1 strip kombu, 3"–4"
2 shiitake mushrooms, soaked and sliced
4 cups water including shiitake soaking water
$\frac{1}{2}$ cube tofu, cut into smaller cubes
3–5 Tbsps. tamari soy sauce
1–2 sheets toasted nori, cut into small pieces
3 chopped scallions

Make a soup stock by bringing kombu, shiitake, and water to a boil, and simmering for 5 minutes. Take out the kombu and shiitake. Boil the tofu cubes and take them out when they rise to the top. Add the tamari and simmer for 5 to 7 minutes. Put in some noodles (only add what you are immediately going to eat and keep the rest aside) until they become warm, then dish them out into individual bowls. Place some tofu, shiitake slices, nori, and scallions on top of each bowl, pour some broth over them and serve.

For variation:

1) Use any combination of shiitake, kombu, or bonito flake soup stocks.
2) Add different kinds of sea vegetables, root, or green vegetables to the broth (they can be left in once they are put in), boil them until they are soft, and add the tamari soy sauce.
3) Add different kinds of sea vegetables, root, green, boiled, sautéed, or raw (thinly sliced) vegetables as a garnish on top. Roasted seeds, fu (soak and boil it in the broth previously as was done with the tofu above), cooked seitan or tempeh, and grated daikon or ginger can also be added.
4) As a general rule, you can add anything as long as there is some kind of sea vegetable present as well as some kind of pungent item in the garnish. This would include scallions, diced raw onions, chives, and grated ginger or daikon. (They help digestion.)

Zaru Soba

> **Soba, previously boiled**
> **1 Tbsp. tamari soy sauce**
> **1 Tbsp. brown rice vinegar**
> **4 Tbsps. kombu soup stock**
> **Chopped scallions**
> **Nori, toasted and cut into thin strips**

Place soba noodles onto an individual serving plate and place a few strips of nori on top. (In Japan they have special individual bamboo serving "plates" which allows soba to drain.) Combine tamari soy sauce, rice vinegar, kombu stock, and scallions into a small bowl to make a dip for the noodles. Make a dip for each person.

2. Seitan is made from the gluten of hard spring or winter whole wheat flours (they contain the most gluten). Seitan is protein-rich.

Seitan

(This can also be bought in natural food stores. Avoid ones that have been heavily spiced if you are healing.)

> **3½ lbs. whole wheat flour (spring or winter)**
> **8–9 cups of water**

Place the flour into a large stainless-steel mixing bowl, gradually add the water, form a dough, and knead it for 5 to 15 minutes until it becomes stiff and earlobe consistency.

Submerge the dough in water and let it sit for 5 to 10 minutes. Then knead and separate the dough in the water until the liquid is full of bran and starch.

Drain the seitan in a colander which you place inside a large pot. (If you want, save the soaking water, starch and bran. It can be used to thicken soups, sauces, stews, puddings, and so on, as well as for pancakes, waffles, and sourdough starter.) Add cold water to the pot and start to knead all the bran out of the gluten.

If this water also becomes overly branny, add fresh water. (You may save this bran water as well, if you like.) One by one, take small pieces of the gluten and wash the bran out of them. You can run them under the tap. (Some remaining flecks of bran here and there is all right. You do not have to worry about trying to get it perfectly bran-free.)

When finished, separate the gluten into several pieces and drop them into a pot of boiling water until they rise to the surface. (Or you can deep-fry them until they puff up and turn golden brown. Try it this way when no longer healing. It is delicious.)

You can cook the seitan further if you want. Put a piece of kombu, seitan, ⅓ to ¼ cup tamari soy sauce, and 6 cups of water into a pot, bring to a boil, turn flame to low, cover, and simmer for about ½ hour. Eat as is or add to other dishes including soups, salads, vegetables, stews, grains, and the like.

Seitan Stew

  2 cups cooked seitan, sliced
  1 strip kombu, soaked and sliced
  1 cup onions, cut into ¼-inch-thick half-moons
  ½ cup celery, cut into ¼-inch-thick diagonals
  1 cup carrots, cut in chunks
  1 to 1½ cups cooked seitan, cut into chunks
  3 to 4 cups kombu-tamari water from cooking seitan
  ½ 1½ cups starch-bran water from cooking seitan, or 1 rounded
     Tbsp. kuzu, dissolved in 1 cup water
  Chopped scallions or parsley for garnish

Put the kombu in a pot. Add the onions, celery, carrots, and seitan. Pour in the kombu-tamari cooking water and bring to a boil. Cover and lower the heat. Simmer until all the vegetables are soft, about 30 to 40 minutes. Add the starch-bran water or kuzu to thicken, and stir well. Let simmer for another 15 to 20 minutes. Garnish with chopped scallions or parsley and serve.

Sweet and Sour Seitan

> 1 cup burdock root, cut in chunks
> 1 cup apple juice
> 3 cups seitan-tamari cooking water
> 3 4 Tbsps. kuzu
> Brown rice vinegar
> ¼ cup chopped scallions

Put the seitan, burdock, apple juice, and seitan cooking water in a pot. Bring to a boil. Cover, and lower the heat to medium-low. Simmer until the burdock is soft. Reduce the heat to low, and add the diluted kuzu and a small amount of brown rice vinegar. Simmer for 2 to 3 minutes. When done, place in a serving bowl and mix in the chopped scallions. Serve hot.

3. Fu is a by-product of wheat gluten. It looks like a cracker and is packaged and available in natural food stores. You can get fu in flat sheets or thick rounds which are available in small or large sizes.

Fu with Vegetables

> 3 to 4 *zenryu* (round) fu, soaked and sliced into thirds
> 1 cup carrots, cut in chunks
> 3 medium onions, cut in chunks
> 10 to 12 Brussels sprouts
> 1 strip kombu, 6″–8″, soaked and cut into small squares
> Tamari soy sauce or miso
> Sea salt

Place kombu in a pan. Group each vegetable separately over kombu. Add approximately ½ inch water and a pinch of sea salt. Cover pot and bring to a boil. Reduce flame to low and simmer ½ hour. Season with tamari soy sauce or 1 teaspoon miso puréed in ¼ cup water. Continue cooking until the liquid is almost evaporated. Gently shake pot, with lid on, to allow seasoning to mix with vegetables. Serves 4.

Fu and Broccoli in Broth

> 1 strip kombu, 6″–8″, soaked
> 4 5 cups water

1 cup fu, soaked and sliced
1 cup broccoli floweretts and stems
Tamari soy sauce

Put the kombu and water in a pot and bring to a boil. Cover
and lower the heat to medium-low. Simmer for about 10 minutes. Remove the kombu, drain, and set aside for future use.
Add the fu to the water and simmer for 5 minutes. Add the
broccoli and simmer until done. The broccoli should be bright
green. When the broccoli is just about done, season with a little
tamari soy sauce, and simmer for 2 to 3 minutes longer.
Transfer to individual serving bowls and serve while hot.

4. Sourdough bread. When healing, it is best to abstain from baked
flour products, as mentioned before, but if you do crave some,
natural, unyeasted sourdough bread is best.
    Yeast is not recommended as it can cause indigestion, and can
weaken the intestines.
    Hard spring or winter wheat flours make the best bread as they
contain much gluten which helps the bread rise. Any other flour
can be added in smaller proportions for a variation in taste, as
can any cooked grains. (Cooked grains that have already gone
sour can replace the sourdough starter.)
    Before making a sourdough bread, you first need to make
a starter.

Sourdough Starter

1 cup whole wheat flour
1–1½ cups well or spring water

Put flour and water into a bowl and mix them into a thick
batter or porridge-like consistency, adding more flour or water
as needed. Cover with a damp towel, and let it sit for 2 to 4
days at room temperature. When it bubbles and becomes sour,
it is ready to use.

Sourdough Bread (2 Loaves)

5 cups whole wheat flour
1 cup sourdough starter (or sour seitan water)
2 cups water
1 tsp. sea salt

Mix the starter, water, and 2½ cups (a half) of the flour, let sit
uncovered in a warm place for an hour or so until it rises.

(At this point, you can save half of this batter for an on-going starter which you can keep using, adding to and recycling every week; the longer it has been around the better the bread. If you do not want to bake one week, mix in a few spoonfuls of flour and water just to keep it going, and to prevent it from spoiling. This should be stored in the refrigerator.)

Add the salt and remaining flour, form into a dough, and on a floured board, start kneading the bread, about 350 to 400 times. The more it is kneaded the better it will rise, as the bread gets more and more elastic, glutenous, and smooth. This is the secret to non-yeasted breads.

Place dough into a lightly oiled bowl, cover with a damp towel, and let it sit overnight at room temperature.

The next morning, punch the dough down, knead it for a few minutes, and divide it in half. Place the halves into a couple of oiled bread pans, and with a knife, make a length-wise slit down the center of the tops. The slit helps to give the bread some room to grow and lets steam escape. Place them in a very warm place and let sit for another 2 to 3 hours, or until the bread rises and the slits begin to open.

Make the slits deeper, and take an oiled rubber spatula and pull the bread away from the sides of the pans. Bake at 350° to 375°F. for about an hour, or until the bread forms a beautiful brown crust.

Insert a chopstick or fork into the bread and pull it out again. If no flour sticks to it, the bread is done. Also, when tapping the bottom, you will hear a hollow sound if the bread is finished. Remove from the pans and let the loaves cool on a bread rack for a couple of hours. Eating the bread while it is still hot may cause an upset stomach. Keep loaves in a cool, dark place, wrapped in a clean cotton cloth or towel.

Slice with a bread knife. If the bread becomes hard, you can steam the slices you want to eat for a few minutes. They then become moist and appear freshly baked.

9. Soups ━━━━━━━━━━━━━━━━━━━━━━━━━━━

The most helpful soups for regular use include:

For All Disorders:

Miso soup with wakame or daikon radish and sweet vegetables
Millet, rice, or barley soup with sweet vegetables

For Obesity:

Tamari broth with shiitake mushrooms

For Anorexia:

Bean soups
Occasionally add pieces of mochi to soups
Squash, carrot, or other sweet-vegetable soups

For Bulimia:

Light tamari broth with shiitake mushrooms, leafy greens and/or
daikon radish
Occasionally season soups with rice or barley vinegar,
umeboshi or lemon juice

Soup at the beginning of a meal prepares the digestive system for all
the following dishes. Just about anything can be put into a soup.
Practically all types of grains, beans and their products, vegetables,
sea vegetables, and occasionally, fish, can be used.

Soups can be adapted seasonally (and be either warming or cooling),
and can add contrast to the rest of the meal. There are some general
guidelines on deciding what kind of soup to use.

In the winter, make more hearty stews and thick soups with more
root vegetables, grains, or beans, and use more salt. In the summer,
make lighter soups with less ingredients and more liquid, more greens,
tofu, and so on. Also make greater use of clear or light tamari-broth
soups in hot weather.

For anorexia, small amounts of pan-fried or broiled mochi may be
added often to soups. Mochi may be made at home or purchased in
a natural food store. It should be cut into small cubes or other shapes,
and placed without oil in a pre-heated pan. Cover and cook until
puffed, then add to soups. This is especially good for miso or broth
soups. You can also create soups with a slightly sweet taste by using
sweet vegetables such as squash, carrots, parsnips, onions, and

cabbage. Depending on the disorder, vegetables may be occasionally sautéed in a small amount of oil before adding them to soups, for extra flavor.

Care should be taken to balance soup with the rest of the meal. Some examples are:

1. Make a bean soup for a light meal lacking in more protein-rich dishes such as beans, tempeh, or natto.

2. Make a sweet-vegetable soup (squash, carrots, parsnips, etc.) if the meal is lacking this sweet taste.

3. Make a root-vegetable soup if the meal is mostly greens and vice versa.

4. Make a grain soup to balance a more light meal.

5. Use finely chopped vegetables if the meal contains all big chunks and vice versa.

6. Use a color in the soup which is not represented in the meal.

7. If you are not making miso soup, you can add miso somewhere else in the meal.

Use a ladle to serve your soups. This can be kept on a plate on the counter next to the soup pot or in a bowl during the course of the meal, ready to be used whenever needed.

Especially during the first few months, it is recommended that everyday, one of your meals should contain miso soup (unless you have soft miso rice that day). Also everyday, at least one of your soups should contain sea vegetables. Garnishes are important (parsley or scallions) to balance your soups, as well as for decoration.

1. *Miso soup:*   Miso is an indispensible part of the macrobiotic diet. It gives vitality, strengthens the digestive system and blood quality, and improves assimilation of carbohydrates. When healing, eat a small amount everyday, particularly in miso soup.

   Miso is very salty so care must be taken to avoid consuming too much of it at one time. To use, add a spoonful of water to a couple of tablespoons or more of miso, and mix it in to make a puree. Then, add this to the soup (or any other dish calling for miso).

   Miso should be added at the end, after all the ingredients have softened, and generally should not be boiled as otherwise valuable healing enzymes are destroyed. However, it is important to note

that the soup must be simmered for a few minutes after the miso is added to help assimilate it into the body. If this is not done, tightness in the body can arise.
The recipes below are for Hatcho (soybean) or mugi (barley) miso.

Basic Miso Soup

Wakame or kombu, soaked and sliced
Choice of vegetables
Pureed miso
Water
Scallion or parsley garnish

Soak wakame or kombu for 10 minutes and slice. Boil the slices in water, cutting your vegetables in the meantime. Add the vegetables to the boiling water and cook until they are soft. Dilute and puree the miso with some of the soup water, turn down the flame, and when the soup has stopped bubbling, gently add and stir the miso puree into the soup. Simmer for 2 to 4 minutes and serve with a garnish. It is important that the soup be light and energetic by keeping your vegetables fresh and crispy, being careful not to overcook them.

Wakame and Daikon Miso Soup

$\frac{1}{2}$ cup wakame, washed, soaked and sliced
$\frac{1}{2}$ cup daikon, cut in half-moons
4 cups spring water
$1\frac{1}{2}$ Tbsps. pureed miso
2 scallions, sliced

Follow the recipe for *Basic Miso Soup*. Serves 6.

Celery Miso Soup

$\frac{1}{2}$ cup celery, cut into 1" pieces
$\frac{1}{2}$ cup thinly sliced onions
1 tsp. dark sesame oil
1 quart spring water
$1\frac{1}{4}$ $1\frac{1}{2}$ Tbsp. miso
1 sheet toasted nori, for garnish

Sauté the celery and onions in the oil. Add enough water or stock to cover the vegetables, and bring to a boil. Add the remaining liquid, cover the pot, and cook until the vegetables become tender. Put the miso in a bowl, add $\frac{1}{4}$ cup of the broth from the pot, and puree. Add the puree to the pot and simmer for a few minutes. Garnish with nori cut in small strips or squares, and serve.

2. *Clear broth or tamari soy sauce soup:* This is a light soup which is very appealing in the hot summer months or when the rest of the meal is more heavy. A stronger tamari broth is very good as a standard supper soup or for noodles.

For a clear soup, make a soup stock (examples are listed at the end of this chapter), and add the vegetables and some form of salt. One way to add variety, in both the flavor and appearance, is to use different salt-based seasonings. Suggestions include:

A. Keep the clear color of the soup stock by using sea salt (a pinch or two for every cup of liquid).

B. Make it darker with 2 to 3 tablespoons of tamari soy sauce for every 4 cups of liquid (most often used).

C. Use 1 tablespoon of umeboshi paste, or 2 to 3 tablespoons of umeboshi vinegar, or 2 to 3 umeboshi plums for every 4 cups of liquid. This gives an attractive pink coloring to your soup.

Tofu, Watercress, Tamari-Broth Soup

1 cube fresh tofu, cut into smaller cubes
1 bunch watercress, washed
½ carrot, cut into very thin matchsticks
1 onion, cut into very thin half-moons
4 cups soup stock
2–3 Tbsps. tamari soy sauce

Bring the soup stock to a boil, drop in the watercress for 2 seconds and then remove, setting it aside to drain for the time being. Add the carrots and onions until they are soft. Then add the tamari and tofu (until it rises to the top) and simmer over a low flame for 3 to 5 minutes. Dish the soup out into individual bowls and garnish with the boiled watercress (which you may chop into more bite-size slices if you desire). Serves 4.

3. *Grain and bean soups:* You can pressure-cook these soups first or just boil them gently for a longer time.

A. Boiling. To boil, layer the vegetables in a pot. Place the more yin vegetables on the bottom and the more yang ones on top (except for greens which are added later and placed on top). Then add the grains or beans, and enough water just to barely cover everything. Bring to a slow boil, adding more water as the grains or beans expand. You can place a heat deflector underneath to help prevent burning. This is the same method used in boiling beans (see *Beans and Bean Products* chapter), except that instead of boiling away the excess liquid in the end, we add more to make it soupy. The salt and/or miso or tamari are added after the grain or bean has softened (simmer another 3 to 10 minutes after the seasoning is added). More water can be added if the consistency is too thick.

Soaking the grain or bean beforehand shortens the cooking time. You can also use previously cooked grains or beans. In this case, first boil the vegetables until they are soft before adding them. Also, you may sauté the vegetables and/or roast the grains or beans beforehand. An optional piece of kombu may be added in the bottom of the pot.

Millet Soup

1 cup carrots, diced
1 cup onions, diced
1 cup millet
Spring water
Sea salt

Rinse millet under cold running water, drain, and pan-roast in a dry pan approximately 10 minutes, or until the millet gives off a nutty aroma. Remove from flame. In a soup pot, layer onions, carrot, and millet from bottom to top. Add spring water just to cover. Bring to a boil, reduce heat, and simmer, covered, 30 minutes, adding more water as the level is reduced. You can vary the consistency of the soup by adding more water toward the end. Season with sea salt, and simmer 2 to 3 minutes more. Garnish with chopped scallions or parsley. Serves 4.

Barley Shiiitake Soup

1 cup barley, soaked 6–8 hours, or overnight
3 shiitake mushrooms, soaked 5–10 minutes
2 pinches sea salt
5–6 cups spring water
A few drops tamari soy sauce to taste

Pressure-cook all ingredients for 40 to 45 minutes. Let the pressure come down completely, and uncover. Bring to a boil again, add tamari soy sauce, turn the flame to low, place a heat deflector underneath, and simmer for another 10 minutes. Serves 4.

B. Pressure-cooking. The grains or beans are first pressure-cooked. The cover is then taken off. Then add the salt (especially in the case of beans, as some grain dishes can take salt from the beginning), tamari soy sauce, or miso, and perhaps some vegetables. Now simmer, up to 20 to 30 minutes longer, depending on the dish.

Chick-Pea Soup

1½ cups cooked chick-peas
1 stalk celery, thinly sliced
½ small head cauliflower, cut in small floweretts
1 leek, thinly sliced
4 pieces dried tofu, soaked 15 minutes and cubed
5–6 cups kombu soup stock
Sea salt
1 sheet toasted nori
Parsley

Bring stock to boil in a soup pot. Add dried, soaked tofu, then celery, leek, cauliflower, and beans. Simmer 30 minutes. Add sea salt to taste. Garnish with toasted nori, cut into thin strips, and parsley. Serves 6.

4. *Soup stocks:* These soup stocks can be used for any of the above types of soups. They are particularly good for the clear, miso, and vegetable soups.

Kombu Soup Stock

1 strip kombu, 3″–6″
5–6 cups spring water

Wipe dust from kombu with a clean, damp cloth. Leave the white powder on. Bring the kombu and water to a boil, simmer about 3 minutes, and remove the kombu. It can be reused for another stock (boil it longer the next time to get more out of it), added to another dish, or sliced and used in this one.
Other variations:

a) 4 shiitake mushrooms, simmer 5–6 minutes
b) 2 Tbsps. bonito fish flakes, simmer 3–4 minutes
c) Any combination of kombu, shiitake, and bonito
d) Odds and ends of vegetables such as onion skins, cabbage cores, roots, tops, and so on. Wash well, boil 5 minutes, and discard or use for compost.
e) Other sea vegetables such as wakame and dulse
f) Dry-roast grains such as rice, sweet rice, millet, buckwheat, or

barley until a nutty fragrance is emitted, and use for stock.
Simmer 4–5 minutes.

g) *Chirimen iriko* (small, whole dried fish available in natural and Oriental food stores). Boil 2 Tbsps. 3–4 minutes.
h) Leftover liquid from boiling vegetables
i) Water left over from cooking beans
j) Diluted water left over from cooking seitan

5. *Vegetable Soups:* Vegetable soups are simple and easy to prepare. They can be made plain by using only one type of vegetable or mixed by combining several vegetables.

Squash Soup

1 medium-sized buttercup, butternut, or Hokkaido squash
4–5 cups spring water
¼–½ tsp. sea salt
Toasted nori, cut into 1″ squares for garnish
Chopped parsley or sliced scallions for garnish

Wash the squash and remove the skin and seeds. Cut the squash into large chunks; you should have about 4 to 5 cups. Put the squash in a pot, and add the water and a pinch of sea salt. Bring to a boil. Cover, lower the heat, and simmer until the squash is soft, about 40 minutes to an hour. Pour the squash and cooking water into a hand food mill and puree. Return the pureed squash to the pot, season with the remaining sea salt, and simmer for several minutes. Pour the soup into individual serving bowls, garnish with a few squares of toasted nori, and serve.

Corn Soup with Kuzu

1½ cups fresh corn kernels
1 small onion, minced
3 cups spring water
1½ Tbsp. kuzu dissolved in ¼ cup water
¼ tsp. sea salt
1½ Tbsp. tamari soy sauce
Toasted nori, cut into 1″ squares for garnish

Make a stock by simmering corn cobs in water for 10 to 15 minutes. Remove cobs. Add corn, onion, and sea salt. Bring to a boil and simmer 15 minutes. Add kuzu and tamari soy sauce and simmer 1 minute more, or until thick. Garnish with nori. Can be served hot or cold. Serves 2 to 3.

10. Vegetables ━━━━━━━━━━

Most helpful dishes for regular use include:

For Obesity:

> **Boiled, steamed, or blanched leafy-green vegetables**
> **Dried daikon with sea vegetables**
> **Nishime-style vegetables, especially daikon**
> **Boiled or pressed salad**

For Anorexia:

> **Nishime-style vegetables, especially made with root and sweet round vegetables, and stews**
> **Kinpira (with oil)**
> **Boiled or steamed leafy-green vegetables**
> **Miso or rice bran pickles**

For Bulimia:

> **Lightly steamed or water-sautéed green vegetables**
> **Boiled or pressed salad**
> **Brine or other light pickles**

As much as possible, get organically grown, chemical-free vegetables. Besides being healthier, they are more delicious. Organic farmers put much care and attention into producing food that benefits both mankind and the planet. Also, avoid dull-colored, limp, yellow-leafed, soft, spotted, or wrinkled items, as they are either too old, spoiled, dried up and/or lacking in vitality.

Choose locally grown produce as often as possible, though in the north during the winter you would have to rely more on southern-grown ones. Prepackaged items tend to spoil more quickly. Stay away from canned and frozen foods. They have no energy and may have added salt, sugar, and preservatives, all of which are best avoided. Also, be careful not to buy waxed items.

At home, immediately remove any yellow leaves and spoiled parts of your vegetables before storing them. This helps to preserve the rest for a longer time. When storing vegetables in the refrigerator, keep them in a paper bag; this allows them to absorb extra moisture and thereby retards spoilage. A plastic bag retains water, does not allow your vegetables to breathe, and causes them to grow soggy and spoil more quickly. Keep vegetables separated from fruits for better preservation.

Do not wash vegetables until you are ready to use them. Any soil left on them helps to keep them fresh longer. When you do wash them, particularly the leafy greens, it helps to submerge them in a big bowl of water. Gently swish them and then wash each leaf individually. This automatically separates and loosens the sand, soil, and dirt which settles to the bottom of the bowl, as the greens stay afloat. This is much more effective and easier than just trying to rinse them under the tap. Roots can be scrubbed gently with a vegetable brush (*tawashi*) to remove the soil, but make sure to keep the skin on. (Do not peel organic vegetables, as they are not sprayed, or covered with wax. The skins contain many nutrients.)

To wash leeks, cut them in half lengthwise, and clean out all the dirt trapped between the layers of leaves. The soil usually collects in the section where the colors change from white to green.

Always use cold water when cleaning vegetables as hot water washes out many vitamins and minerals. Wash vegetables quickly. Soaking for any length of time also depletes valuable nutrients.

Within one dish, cut your vegetables uniformly for even cooking. Within a meal, have a variety of different sizes represented in several dishes—smaller for sautéed items, and bigger chunks for stews, for example.

Save the tops and roots of vegetables. They can be cleaned, chopped very finely, and incorporated into vegetable dishes. You can also leave them uncut and use them in a soup stock. Using the whole plant helps to create a balance in your system.

I recommend the square, Japanese vegetable knives (see *Cookware* chapter) for cutting vegetables. They are very handy, flexible, and easy to use. With these knives, we do not cut straight down, or use them like a saw. Starting with the front tip or edge, gently slide the length of the blade across your vegetables in one smooth stroke. *Important: Always Keep Your Fingertips Curled Underneath So That Your Knuckles Show When You Are Cutting.* This helps to protect the fingers from accidental cuts and slips, and allows a better grip on the vegetable as well.

There are several cutting styles to choose from. Here is a partial listing.

1)	**Round slices**	4)	**Rectangles**
2)	**Diagonal slices**	5)	**Half-moons**
3)	**Triangular shapes**	6)	**Quarters**

7) Matchsticks
8) Cubing, dicing, and mincing
9) Shavings

10) Slicing cabbages
11) Slicing big leafy greens
12) Wedge slices

Fig. 19 Vegetable Cutting Styles

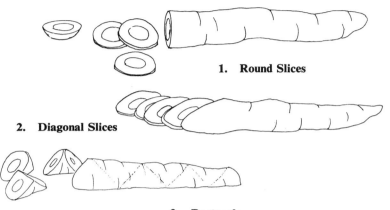

1. Round Slices

2. Diagonal Slices

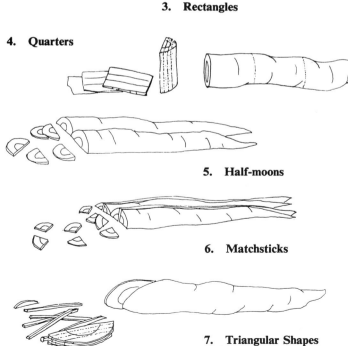

3. Rectangles

4. Quarters

5. Half-moons

6. Matchsticks

7. Triangular Shapes

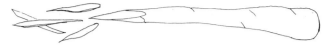

8. Shavings

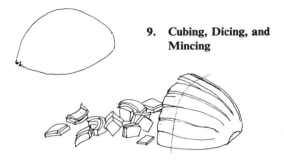

9. Cubing, Dicing, and Mincing

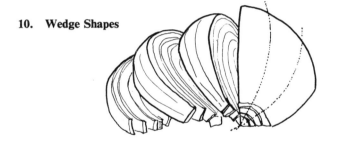

10. Wedge Shapes

11. Slicing Cabbages

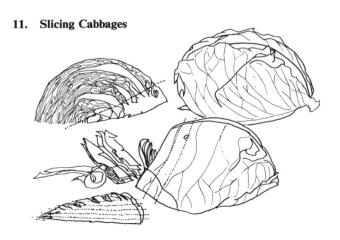

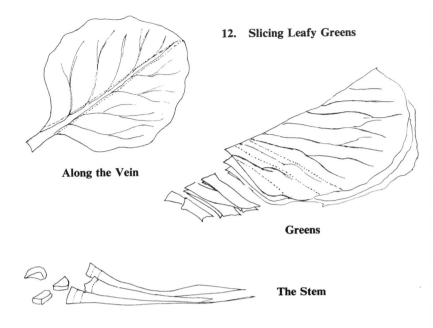

12. Slicing Leafy Greens

Along the Vein

Greens

The Stem

Include a variety of different kinds of vegetables (roots, greens, round vegetables, and sea vegetables, for example) in a meal, as well as an assortment of textures and colors. Also, use a variety of cooking styles. Here are some of the main methods that we use.

1. *Boiling methods:* There are two main styles: quick, short-time boiling and slow, longer-time boiling. You can have some kind of boiled vegetable at nearly every meal.

    A. Quick boiling (blanching): Blanching is the best way to cook leafy green vegetables. Fill a pot with 1 to 2 inches of water and bring to a boil. Dip in vegetables and take them out quickly. An oil skimmer lifts them easily. Drain the vegetables in a colander. (Place a plate underneath to catch any excess liquid. This water can be put back into the pot.)

    The main point in this style is to cook in as short a time as possible, retaining crispness and bright colors. For example, watercress can be taken out after 15 to 30 seconds. Others take a little longer, in varying degrees, but not that much more. Kale, mustard greens, collard greens, cabbage,

Chinese cabbage, broccoli, cauliflower, celery, and others can be used.

A pinch of salt in the water helps retain bright colors (but leave it out when cooking bitter vegetables such as watercress and mustard greens, as salt will hold in the bitter flavor).

Root vegetables can also be cooked in this way but you have to cut them into very thin slices. Boil them for a slightly longer time than you would with greens.

If you want to boil several different vegetables, do them one by one. Start with the lighter-tasting varieties like the cabbages, and end with more strong-tasting ones like mustard greens, so that the flavor of the latter will not overpower the flavor of the former. Each vegetable's distinct individuality should be maintained.

You can use the leftover boiling water as a base for a soup. Or you can add some kuzu to it (2 teaspoons for one cup water) to thicken it into a sauce to pour over your vegetables. To do this, first dilute the kuzu in a small amount of cold water. Turn the flame to low under the boiled water and pour the kuzu in. Stir and simmer until the liquid turns clear. Add a little tamari soy sauce or umeboshi paste to taste, and pour this over boiled vegetables.

Two recipe examples:

Boiled Broccoli and Cauliflower

2 cups broccoli floweretts and stems
2 cups cauliflower floweretts and stems
4 cups spring water

Boil water. Add the cauliflower, cover, and boil until it is done, about 5 minutes. The cauliflower should be soft but not so cooked that it falls apart. Remove the cauliflower and transfer it to a bowl. Add broccoli to the same water and boil for 3 to 4 minutes, or until done. It should be bright green when cooked.

Remove the broccoli and arrange it in the bowl so that the cauliflower is surrounded by a ring of bright green broccoli. If desired, a thin sauce of water, tamari soy sauce, grated fresh ginger, and fresh lemon juice can be poured over the vegetables.

Boiled Salad

8–10 Chinese cabbage leaves, cut into 1″ slices
2 cups onions, cut into half-moons

1 cup celery, sliced thinly on the diagonal
1 cup carrots, cut into matchsticks
4 cups spring water
2 Tbsps. tamari soy sauce
$\frac{1}{4}$ tsp. grated fresh ginger
2 Tbsps. roasted sesame seeds

Boil water. Quickly and separately boil the Chinese cabbage, carrots, onions, and celery. Drain each and mix them together into a serving bowl. Prepare a dressing by combining the tamari soy sauce, 2 to 3 tablespoons spring water, and the grated ginger. Mix the ingredients together and pour over vegetables. Add the roasted sesame seeds and mix everything together before serving.

B. Slow, longer-time boiling: This style is basically for root vegetables such as daikon, carrots, onions, lotus root, burdock, and so on, as well as squash. This style gives a calming but strong and healing energy.

One or two pieces of kombu are usually placed in the bottom of the pot to help prevent the vegetables from burning, to add extra minerals and flavor, and to help harmonize all the ingredients.

The vegetables are then layered on top of the kombu, with the more yin ones on the bottom and the more yang ones on the top. The yin rising energy meets the yang descending energy and the dish is better integrated.

If the vegetables are fairly dry, put in enough water to just cover them. If they are fresh and more watery, cover them only halfway with water. Add a pinch of salt, cover the pot, bring everything to a boil, turn the flame to low, and simmer for about 20 minutes, or until soft. The time depends on the type, quality, and slice sizes of the vegetables used. Do not mix or stir the vegetables. When the vegetables are soft, add some tamari soy sauce for more flavor, and simmer another 5 minutes. Shiitake mushrooms, dried tofu, tempeh, and seitan may also be added to this dish.

Daikon, Lotus Root, and Shiitake Mushrooms

1 daikon, sliced into $\frac{3}{4}''$ rounds
3 shiitake mushrooms, soaked
1 lotus root, sliced into $\frac{1}{4}''$ rounds
1 piece kombu

1 pinch sea salt
Enough water to just cover the vegetables
Tamari soy sauce to taste

Place kombu in the bottom of the pot. Add the other ingredients in this order from the bottom up: shiitake, daikon, and lotus root. Add water and sea salt, cover, and follow the above directions. Serves 3.

Whole Onions in Miso

6 whole medium-sliced onions, peeled
1 to 2 strips kombu, 8″, soaked 4–5 minutes
Spring water
1 1½ Tbsps. miso
Optional: 1 2 tsps. kuzu
Finely chopped parsley

Make 6 to 8 shallow cuts in each onion to give it the appearance of being sectioned, but do not cut too deeply. The slices will allow the onions to open up like flowers while they are cooking. Put the whole onions on top of the kombu in a pot. Add water to half cover the onions. Pour miso pureed in a little water on top of the onions. Cover the pot, and bring to a boil. Lower the heat, and simmer until the onions are soft and translucent, about 30 minutes. If there is too much liquid remaining in the pot, thicken with kuzu after removing the onions. Pour the kuzu sauce or the plain cooking liquid over the onions. Garnish with chopped parsley. Serves 6.

2. *Nishime style:* This is a medicinal form of cooking using a minimal amount of water. For this you need a heavy pot with a heavy lid, or some cookware specifically designed for waterless cooking.

   Kombu at the bottom of the pot helps to prevent burning, as well as adding extra minerals and taste.

   Root vegetables such as carrots, daikon, turnips, burdock, lotus root, onions, and hard winter squash (acorn, buttercup, or Hokkaido), cabbage, and shiitake mushrooms are normally used. They are usually cut into 2-inch chunks (except for burdock which is cut about half the size or smaller), and layered on top of the kombu from yin to yang (yin on the bottom). Squash dissolves and loses its shape if cooked for a long time, so you may add it a little later on.

   To cook, soak a piece of kombu until it is soft, cut it into

1-inch squares, and place it in the bottom of a pot. Add enough water just to cover the kombu if the vegetables are fresh and watery. If they are more dry or if using burdock or losut root, add enough water to cover the vegetables halfway. Put in the vegetables and sprinkle a small amount of sea salt or tamari soy sauce over them.

Cover, set the flame on high until a steam is produced. Then lower the flame and let the vegetables simmer peacefully for 15 to 20 minutes. If water should evaporate during cooking, add a little more to the bottom of the pot if it is necessary to prevent burning.

When all the vegetables have softened, add a few more drops of tamari soy sauce to taste.

Then, replace the cover, and cook over a low flame for 2 to 5 minutes more. After turning off the flame, remove the cover and let the vegetables sit for about 2 minutes. Serve the juice along with the vegetables as it is very delicious.

Tempeh, Squash, and Cabbage Nishime

8 ozs. tempeh
1 small buttercup or other winter squash, cut in large chunks
1 small head green cabbage, cut in large wedges
1 strip kombu, 6"–8", soaked and sliced into 1" pieces
2 pinches sea salt
Tamari soy sauce to taste
Enough water to cover vegetables halfway

Dry-roast tempeh whole until slightly browned on both sides. Cut into small squares. Follow the above directions, adding tempeh on top of cabbage and squash. Serves 6.

A few variation examples:

1) Carrots, cabbage, burdock, kombu
2) Carrots, onion, kombu
3) Carrots, lotus root, burdock, kombu
4) Daikon, shiitake mushrooms, kombu
5) Daikon, lotus root, dried tofu, kombu
6) Parsnips, onions, kombu

Daikon/Daikon Greens

Daikon roots and leaves
1 strip kombu, 3"–6", soaked and sliced
Miso or tamari soy sauce to taste
Enough water to just cover the kombu

Wash and finely slice the daikon roots and leaves. Put the kombu in a pot with enough water to just cover it. Add the roots, cover, and cook with a high steam for 10 minutes or longer. Towards the end, add the leaves, miso or tamari soy sauce to taste and simmer for another 2 to 4 minutes. Other variations (finely chopped):

1) **Turnip and its leaves**
2) **Carrot and its tops (slice tops extra fine)**
3) **Radish and its tops**
4) **Dandelion root and leaves**

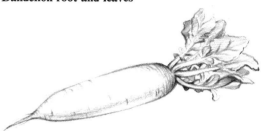

Fig. 20   Daikon Radish

3. *Sautéing:*   There are two ways to sauté: with or without oil, using water as a substitute. When limiting your use of oil, you can use the water-sautéing method as often as you like.

With oil. It is best to use only sesame oil (particularly the dark or roasted variety), and to spread it onto the bottom of a heated pan rather than to pour it in. Put your oil into a cast-iron skillet (do not use too much, perhaps 1 tablespoon for 8 people), and heat it up with a medium-high flame. When the oil seems warm, test it by dropping in one slice of a vegetable. If the oil sizzles, then it is ready, and you can put in the rest of the ingredients.

When water sautéing, simply add a tablespoon or two of water as needed in cooking to prevent burning.

As an option, if using onions, many people like to sauté them first. I find that first sautéing onions, until they become translucent, before putting in the next vegetable (move the onions on top of them), makes a very sweet dish.

Either add the different kinds of vegetables one by one, starting with the ones that take the longest time to cook and ending with the faster-cooking ones; or cut them so that the different types of vegetables will cook at the same rate (soft vegetables in larger slices, tougher ones in thinner slices), and layer them from yin to yang (yin in the bottom).

After putting in the vegetables, add a pinch or two of sea salt. Salt brings out the natural sweetness, draws out the water, and helps to soften the vegetables quicker (it has the opposite effect on grains and beans and is therefore added later on in their case). Gently stir from time to time (with a wooden spoon or cooking chopsticks) to prevent burning.

After about 5 minutes turn the flame to low, cover (unless you are working with really watery items such as Chinese cabbage or tofu), and simmer until the vegetables are soft. The time it takes depends on what is being cooked and the size of your slices. You may need to add a little water to avoid burning, especially when cooking with something like burdock. Add a little soy sauce (and some grated ginger if you wish) at the end for more flavor, and simmer another 2 to 3 minutes. Uncover and boil away any excess water if there is any.

Any vegetable can be sautéed (cut your root vegetables into very thin slices or shavings), as can tofu and tempeh.

Two recipe examples:

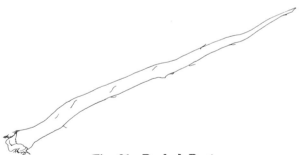

Fig. 21   Burdock Root

Carrot and Burdock Kinpira

(This dish is very strengthening and can be used once or twice a week for those trying to regain vitality. When preparing this dish for persons who must limit their oil intake, substitute the oil with a little water.)

1 cup shaved burdock
2 cups shaved carrots
Optional: dark sesame oil
1 pinch sea salt
Tamari soy sauce to taste
Optional: ½ tsp. grated ginger
Water, if needed to prevent burning
A few parsley sprigs

Heat oil in a skillet, add carrots, burdock, and salt, and follow
the above directions. Add a small amount of water if needed
to prevent burning. Garnish with the parsley. Serves 4 to 6.

Sautéed Vegetables with Tofu

(This type of lighter dish, using some of the "occasional use"
vegetables, is very nice for variety and freshness.)

2 celery stalks, cut into thin diagonal slices
2 carrots, cut into thin diagonal slices
1 medium summer squash, cut into thin diagonal slices
1 cake tofu, cut into 1″ cubes
Dark sesame oil or 1–2 Tbsps. water
1 pinch sea salt
Tamari soy sauce to taste
A dash of grated ginger

Heat oil or water in a skillet, sauté tofu, then celery, carrots,
and squash. Add sea salt. Do not cover. Boil off any excess
liquid. Add tamari soy sauce to taste and simmer another
3 minutes. Add a dash of ginger and serve. Serves 3 to 4.

4. *Pressure-cooking:* This is good for big chunks of root vegetables
and squash (but do not cook greens this way). Use this style as
often as you wish as long as you make sure that you are also
making fresher vegetables such as salad and boiled or steamed
greens to balance all the pressure-cooking that you will be doing
with your grains and beans. After the pressure comes up, carrots
and onions may be done in 5 minutes, and big chunks of lotus
root and burdock in 15 to 20 minutes.

After putting your ingredients into the pressure cooker, add
enough water to just cover the bottom of the pot, approximately
½ to 1 inch. Add salt, cover, bring to pressure over a medium-
high flame. When pressure is up, turn the flame to low and simmer until done. Rinse the pot under cold water if you want to

bring the pressure down quickly. (Do not uncover the pot until the pressure is completely down.)

Pressure-Cooked Carrots, Parsnips, and Onions

2 medium carrots, cut in large chunks
2 medium parsnips, cut in large chunks
2 medium onions, quartered
1 piece kombu
1 pinch sea salt
Enough water to cover the bottom of the pot

Put the kombu in the bottom of the pressure cooker and then add the carrots, parsnips, onions, sea salt, and water. Follow the above directions. Simmer for 5 minutes. Serves 4.

Other variations

1) Other root vegetables, such as daikon, lotus root, burdock, etc.
2) Buttercup or Hokkaido squash
3) Add dried tofu, seitan, dried daikon, or round fu

5. *Steaming:* You can use this method fairly often if you like. To steam, add ½ to 1 inch of cold water in the bottom of a pot, insert a steamer, place your vegetable inside with a pinch of salt, cover, and bring the water to a boil. Then steam for 3 to 10 minutes or more, until your vegetable is soft.

Steaming is good for any kind of vegetable and makes a nice variation to boiling. Be careful not to overcook vegetables. Remove them while they are still crisp and brightly colored.

Steam each kind of vegetable separately unless you are going to serve them mixed together and they take the same amount of time to cook. When you put in a new vegetable, let the water cool a bit so that the vegetable gets cooked more evenly. To keep their bright color, run the vegetables under cold water, and do not cover them until they cool off. The leftover water can be used as soup stock or sauce (just like the boiling water). Steaming is a great way to heat up leftovers, especially rice.

Steamed Collard Greens with Tamari-Vinegar Sauce

3 cups thinly sliced collard greens
Spring water
Tamari soy sauce
Brown rice vinegar

Put a small amount of water in a pot and bring to a boil. Put a steamer in the pot. Set the collards in the steamer and steam for several minutes, or until done. The greens should be bright green and slightly crisp. Remove them and put them in a serving dish. Mix a small amount of tamari soy sauce, brown rice vinegar, and water together to make a sauce. Pour 1 teaspoon of sauce over each serving of collard greens.

6. *Salad:* There are three types of salads:

A. *Boiled Salad:* Refer to the section on boiled vegetables for directions and an example. This can be taken several times a week.

B. *Pressed salad:* This can generally be eaten every two or three days. The vegetables are raw but pressing them with salt helps to yangize them. However, it may still be a little too yin for frequent use in cold weather. In this case, take this only once a week.

To prepare, cut your vegetables into very thin slices, or shred them, and put them in a pickle press with sea salt for one or more hours. Drain off the excess water, wash off the excess salt, and serve. If you do not have a pickle press you can put your vegetables in a bowl and cover them with a plate. Put a rock or some kind of weight (such as a large glass jar filled with water) on top of the plate and press.

Red Cabbage in Umeboshi Vinegar

¼ **red cabbage, shredded**
½ **cup umeboshi vinegar**

Mix ingredients in a pickle press and let sit for approximately 1 hour. If too salty, quickly rinse in cold water before serving.

C. *Regular raw salad:* Persons trying to alleviate obesity should avoid this for a while, perhaps several months. Otherwise, this is recommended about once or twice a week, or more during the hot summer months.

Use the usual salad vegetables such as lettuce, cucumbers, sprouts, carrots, onions, celery, parsley, and so on, but avoid peppers, potatoes, tomatoes, eggplants, and mushrooms. You can also add roasted sesame and pumpkin seeds, whole wheat-bread croutons, cooked chick-peas, pinto beans, rice, bulghur, couscous, noodles, macaroni, wakame, dried dulse, and cooked hijiki, arame, tofu, tempeh, and seitan. Of course, your combinations should be tasteful. Obviously, not all those ingredients are compatible with one another.

Garden Salad

1 ear of corn, kernels removed
1 head lettuce
5–6 red radishes, thinly sliced
1 cucumber, sliced into thin rounds
1 box alfalfa sprouts
1 carrot, shredded

Boil the corn kernels in about ¼ inch of water in a saucepan for 2 to 3 minutes. Set aside kernels to cool. Arrange the lettuce attractively on a serving plate. A nice soft variety, such as Boston lettuce, opens up easily and the leaves can be torn by hand.

Distribute the sliced radishes and cucumbers evenly in a circle on the lettuce leaves. Place the sprouts in small groupings in the center of the circle on top of the lettuce, or around the outside edge, or both. Sprinkle corn kernels over the salad. Finally, add the shredded carrot to the very top of the salad and, if you like, in the cardinal directions.

Serve with a separate sauce, such as umeboshi-plum dressing with a little onion and sesame seeds, tofu dressing with a little umeboshi, a miso-brown-rice-vinegar dressing with a little mirin, or a tamari-ginger dressing with a little mirin.

Tempeh-Macaroni Salad

Spring water
1 lb. tempeh, cut into 1″ squares
Tamari soy sauce
Brown rice vinegar
1 lb. whole wheat macaroni noodles or pasta shells made with artichoke flour
½ head lettuce
½ head cabbage
1 bunch watercress
Parsley springs for garnish

Put about 1 inch of water in a saucepan and add the tempeh squares. Bring to a boil, lower the heat, and cook 20 to 30 minutes until soft. Drain the tempeh and allow it to cool. Prepare a marinade of half tamari soy sauce and half brown rice vinegar using several tablespoons of each. Pour the mixture over the tempeh.

While the tempeh is marinating, boil macaroni until done. Slice lettuce and cabbage or tear by hand into bite-sized pieces. Dip watercress into boiling water for 20 to 30 seconds to remove its bitter taste, or use raw and cut it into small pieces. Mix the pasta, tempeh, and vegetables together very well, and garnish with parsley sprigs.

7. *Baked:*   Baking takes a longer time to cook foods but it gives strength and extra flavor. It is best to bake once in a while for variety rather than on a daily basis.

This style is good for squashes and root vegetables. You can leave them whole (burdock should be sliced), or cut them in half or in chunks.

You can bake them with or without oil, using a casserole dish or a cookie sheet covered with foil. If your vegetables are fresh and juicy you may not need to add water, especially if you oil the sheet or dish and have a good cover. If you do not use oil, add just a little water to cover the suface. If your vegetables are more dried out or are tough, add about a ¼ to ½ inch of water. Adding a dash of salt helps to draw out the water in the vegetables.

Place your vegetables, salt, water, and/or oil into a dish or onto a sheet, cover, turn to 350° to 375°F., and bake for 45 to 60 minutes, or until they are soft. Towards the end you can uncover, let any extra water evaporate, add tamari soy sauce, miso, or some sauce to taste, and simmer for another 5 minutes or so until done.

You can bake squash whole and uncovered on an oiled cookie sheet (with stuffing inside if you prefer). Or you can cut it in half and place the halves on the sheet (again uncovered) with the inside facing down. Do not forget to take out the seeds.

Baked Summer Squash with Miso-Ginger Sauce

    2–3 medium-sized summer squash
    Dark sesame oil
    1 tsp. barley miso
    ¼ tsp. grated fresh ginger
    Spring water
    Parsley sprigs for garnish

Wash the summer squash and slice them in half lengthwise. Slice off the stem ends. Using a knife, make light diagonal slashes in the skin of the squash like this: / / / /. Then make shallow diagonal slices in the opposite direction to create a crisscross effect like this: × × × ×. Oil a baking dish or baking sheet and also lightly oil the skin of the squash. Put the squash on the oiled dish. Bake for about 20 minutes in a pre-heated 375°F. oven.

Put the miso in a suribachi and add the ginger. Puree, adding a small amount of water to make a smooth, creamy sauce. Lightly brush the miso-ginger sauce on top of the squash slices and bake for about 10 to 15 minutes longer. Remove from the oven and arrange the slices on a platter. Garnish with sprigs of parsley. The slices can be cut into 2- to 3-inch lengths before serving.

8. *Pickles:* Pickles are an extremely important addition to your diet. Have a small amount on the side at every meal or at least once a day and eat them with your grains. They aid in digestion, strengthen the intestinal flora, stimulate appetite, and add zest to the meal.

Always use fresh, firm, and crisp vegetables for making pickles. Also, it is imperative that the vegetables, containers, and anything else used for pickling, be thoroughly cleaned. This is done to prevent any unknown substances interacting with the pickling process. For tougher vegetables, it is helpful to quickly blanch them in boiling water before pickling them.

Pickling time ranges from a couple of hours to several months. The main factors influencing pickling time are the size of your vegetables and the amount of salt you use. Small, thinly sliced pieces can be pickled very quickly whereas large, thick, or whole pieces take a long time. Long-time pickling requires more salt to prevent spoiling. You can dip your vegetables in hot boiling water before you pickle them if you choose, especially with largely sliced and/or hard vegetables. This removes the raw flavor and brings out a sweeter taste.

Experimentation may be needed to get the feel of the right amount of salt to use. If the vegetables spoil before they pickle, and/or not much water comes out (for methods that require that it does), there is not enough salt. If too much salt is added, the pickles will become too salty and any other flavor that the vegetables may have had will be covered up. To remove excess salt, rinse or soak your pickles for a little while before you eat them.

If mold starts to form anywhere, take it out immediately so that the rest of the contents will not be affected.

Cover the whole thing with a cheesecloth. It helps to keep dirt and dust out of the pickles while letting the air circulate and enabling them to breathe. (Do not cover with an airtight lid.)

We usually use four main types of pickling methods.

1. *Pressed pickles:* You can make them quickly, in a couple of hours, or you can make them in several weeks.

   A. *Quick pickles:* When pickling for a few hours up to a day or two, you can use a pickle press. But since most of them are made out of plastic, it is not safe to use them for a longer period of time as the poisonous toxic substances in them will start to seep into the vegetables. If you do not have a press or if you want to use something safer, you can take a small glass bowl and find a saucer that fits into it. It should cover the inside as much as possible but still remain loose so that water can escape over the sides. For a weight, you can use a glass jar full of water, grains, or beans, or some clean stones.

   Soft, watery vegetables like thinly sliced cucumbers and very thin matchstick daikon strips can be done in 2 to 3 hours. Other pickles can be made in the morning and be either eaten for dinner or left for 2 to 3 days longer. Some (like harder, less watery vegetables like turnips) may need the extra days. Again, pickling time depends on the size and moisture content of the pieces.

   Vegetables have to be cut into really thin slices or shredded for quick pickling. (An exception is mustard greens which can be made whole and cut when you want to eat them. Mix the salt in really well and wait 2 to 3 days.) Chinese cabbage, red and white cabbage, daikon and its greens, turnips and its greens, celery, radishes, onions, cucumbers and bok choy are good to use. For best results, use only one kind of vegetable at a time. You can add a strip of kombu (perhaps 3 to 6 inches long for two cups of vegetables) for extra minerals and a different flavor. Soak the kombu until it is soft, slice it into thin strips, and put it underneath the vegetables. Grated ginger can be added if you wish.

   For 2 cups of vegetables add about 1 to 2 teaspoons of salt. Mix them together thoroughly. The salt can be substituted with 2 to 4 tablespoons of umeboshi vinegar, paste, or plums and/or shiso leaves. You can also use 2 to 4 tablespoons of soy sauce. Water will start to rise above the saucer or pressure plate. If there is a lot, you can take a little out, but always leave some covering the plate. Cover with a cheesecloth (not necessary if using a press, of course) and wait till it is done.

Onion Pickles

2 cups thinly sliced onions
2–4 Tbsp. tamari soy sauce

Pickle the onions in soy sauce following the above directions. If the onions were cut thinly, they will be done in 2 hours. You can also eat them the next day.

B. *Longer-time pressed pickles:* A wooden keg or ceramic crock are good containers to use for this. A heavy stone or large jar filled with water is placed on top of a plate or a wooden disc, which fits inside, for pressure. Cover the whole thing with a cheesecloth and place in a cool, dark place. Check regularly for mold and remove it immediately if any appears. Sauerkraut is made this way. Below is a sample recipe.

Chinese Cabbage Pickles

1 head Chinese cabbage
Sea salt

Remove the cabbage leaves individually and wash them. Put them in a colander or allow to drain in a dish drainer. When the vegetable has dried, sprinkle a thin layer of sea salt in the bottom of a wooden keg or ceramic crock. Layer the whole cabbage leaves and several pinches of sea salt in the keg or crock, alternating between the salt and cabbage.

The bottom and top layers in the keg or crock should always be salt. Rotate each layer of leaves 90 degrees from the previous layer, for example, from 12 o'clock, to 3 o'clock to 6 o'clock to 9 o'clock. A whole strip of kombu may be added to the bottom of the keg or crock. The kombu absorbs water, adds minerals, and gives its flavor to the pickles.

Place a wooden disc or plate on top of the last layer of cabbage and sea salt. Place several clean heavy rocks or other heavy weight on top of the plate or disc to press the leaves down. If water does not start to come out of the cabbage leaves within 10 to 20 hours, more sea salt is needed. The pickles will spoil if not enough salt or pressure is used.

Check the pickles daily for signs of spoilage. When the water rises to the level of the disc or plate, remove some of the rocks or weights. The water should always just slightly cover the disc or plate. However, do not discard surfacing water, or mold will form, and the pickles will spoil if it spreads. The pickles should be ready to eat in 3 to 4 days, or may be left for several more days for a more sour taste. Store in a cool, dark place. If too salty, rinse under cold water and slice before using. Refrigerated, pickles will keep 1 to 2 months.

2. *Brine pickles:* To make brine pickles, tightly stuff some vegetables into a glass jar. Boil some kind of a brine mixture (see following recipes), let it cool off, and pour it into the jar, filling it up. Cover the top with cheesecloth which you can fasten down with a rubber band, and pickle for several days. When done, store in a refrigerator. This is how dill pickles are made. You can use cucumbers, onions, turnips, rutabagas, daikon, carrots, broccoli, cauliflower, cabbages, greens, and so on.

There are several kinds of brine that you can choose to use, examples of which are presented below. You can use a soup stock if you want. You can add ginger, kombu, shiitake mushrooms, lemon juice and rinds, shiso leaves, grated raw apple, and so on, for extra flavor. Some *ame* rice syrup can be boiled and dissolved into the brine (good with the tamari-based one) for a sweet taste.

Daikon and Carrot Pickles (Salt-Based Brine)

1 daikon, cut in half-moons
2–3 carrots, cut on the diagonal
6 cups spring water
½ cup sea salt
1 strip kombu, 3″, soaked and thinly sliced into strips

Bring water and salt to a boil. Turn the flame to medium-low and simmer until all the salt has dissolved. Let brine cool. Place kombu in the bottom of a glass jar and cover with daikon and carrots. Pour in the cooled brine and fill to the top. Cover with a cheesecloth and keep in a dark location for 3 to 4 days. When finished, keep in the refrigerator.

Red Radish Pickles (Umeboshi Based)

1 cup sliced red radishes
2 3 umeboshi plums

Put the radishes in a pickle press or bowl. You can use the radish greens in this recipe if they are in good condition; wash them and layer them over the radish slices. Break apart the umeboshi with your hands and add the pieces to the radishes. The pits are very strong and may be included, but be sure to remove them before serving. Let sit for several hours or overnight.

Variation: Instead of whole plums, 2 to 3 teaspoons of umeboshi paste or ½ cup of umeboshi vinegar mixed with ¾ cup spring water may be used.

3. *Miso pickles:* Miso pickles are especially helpful for recovering good digestive strength. They are simple to make. Just quickly blanch your vegetables in boiling water, and then submerge and surround them totally in miso. This is used for root vegetables such as carrots, burdock, daikon, turnips, parsnips, and ginger. Broccoli stems make great pickles as well. Greens are too watery.

The vegetables have to be dried until you can bend them like rubber before you put them into the miso. Otherwise, the miso will get too watery and the pickling will not work.

Pickling time depends on the vegetables you use and the size of your slices. Very thin ones can pickle in 3 to 4 days, up to a week. Whole vegetables with slits in their sides can take 1 to 2 weeks, thick slices about 3 months, and whole vegetables (unslitted) can be left in the miso up to a year. Just make sure they are totally submerged (top, bottom, and sides). You do not need to use any pressure.

When the pickles are done, just take them out, rinse them off, slice, and eat them.

Scallion-Miso Pickles

1 bunch scallions
Miso

Wash the scallions and put them in a jar so they are completely covered with miso. Let sit for 1 to 2 days. Remove, scrape off most of the miso, and save it for cooking. Slice the scallions, rinse if too salty, and serve.

Broccoli Stem Miso Pickles

Broccoli stems
A container of miso

Peel leftover broccoli stems unless the skins are soft, quickly
blanch them in boiling water, and submerge them into the
miso for 1 to 2 weeks, depending on how thick they are. You
can leave the skins on if you like. The pickling time will be
much longer then, maybe a month or more. Cover with
a cheesecloth and keep in a cool, dark place until they are done.

4. *Bran pickles:* Bran pickling uses a mixture of bran (rice or
wheat) or rice flour, and sea salt. Like miso pickles, bran pickles
are especially good for weak intestines.

   Quickly dry-roast the bran or flour in a skillet over a medium-
low flame until a nutty fragrance is emitted. Remove from the
skillet and allow it to cool.

   Firm, root vegetables pickle best, but you can also use greens.
The vegetables should all be dried before you use them. A few
hours under the sun works nicely. Daikon, carrots, and parsnips are best when dried longer (several days), until they bend
like rubber.

   A ceramic crock or wooden keg again are the best containers
to use. Cover the pickles with a cheesecloth and keep in a cool,
dark place.

   There are two ways to make bran pickles.

A. *Bran pickles A:* Boil some salt and water, let it cool off,
place in a crock or keg, and thoroughly mix in the roasted bran
or flour to form a paste. Take your dried vegetables and totally
submerge them into this paste making sure that the vegetables
are not touching each other. Pack this whole thing down until
it is firm and solid. Cover with a cheesecloth.

   If you slice the vegetables into fairly small pieces they will be
done in a week or two. You can also leave them whole. Whole
root vegetables can take as long as 3 to 5 months to pickle.
Add more salt if you want to pickle for a long time. (Whole
leaves take only a couple of weeks.)

   As you remove your finished pickles, you can keep adding
new vegetables. When you do, add more bran and salt. Mix the
paste once in a while. If kept well, you can use this paste for
years as you add and subtract vegetables from it.

Short-Time Paste Proportions (1–2 Weeks)

10–12 cups bran or rice flour
¼–¼ cup sea salt
3–5 cups water

Longer-Time Paste Proportions (Up to 3–5 Months)

10–12 cups bran or rice flour
1½–2 cups sea salt
3–5 cups water

B. *Bran pickles B:* This method is made by alternating layers of vegetables with layers of the bran and sea salt mixture.

Mix roasted bran with sea salt and cover the bottom of a crock or keg. Then, add a layer of dried vegetables. Add another layer of bran and salt. Keep alternating. The last layer should be bran. Insert a plate or a wooden disc into the crock on top of the mixture, place a heavy weight on top of the plate, and press the whole thing. The plate or disc should be loose fitting but wide enough to cover the contents as much as possible. A clean stone or a jar filled with water can be used as a weight. Cover with a cheesecloth and put in a cool, dark place. When water begins to rise, lighten the weight. When pickles are done, rinse off the bran, slice, and eat.

Just as in *Bran pickles A*, you can either slice the vegetables into fairly small pieces or leave them whole. As before, whole pieces take a much longer time to pickle and require more salt.

● Short-Time Proportions (1–2 Weeks)

10–12 cups bran or rice flour
⅛–¼ cups sea salt

● Longer-Time Proportions (3–5 Months)

10–12 cups bran or rice flour
1½–2 cups sea salt

Chinese Cabbage Bran Pickles

2 heads Chinese cabbage
Bran & salt using shorter-time proportions

Separate the individual leaves from the body of the cabbage. Wash, they dry the leaves for two days, preferably under the sun. Make alternating layers of cabbage with sea salt (the bottom and top layers should be salt), and place a plate and heavy weight on top. Water should rise to the level of the plate in 10 hours. If not, add more weight and/or a little more salt.

When the water has risen, drain it out thoroughly. Then relayer the cabbage alternating it with the bran. (The bottom and top layers should be bran.) Replace the weight.

The pickles should be ready in a week. When done, wash out the bran, slice, and serve. (The reason for draining out the water first is to produce a less salty and more sweet-tasting pickle. Also, the Chinese cabbage is a pretty watery vegetable. Other vegetables can be layered in one step, using the bran the first time around, as mentioned before this recipe.)

11. Beans and Bean Products ▬▬▬

Most helpful dishes include:
For All Disorders:

Azuki beans with squash or other sweet vegetables
Tofu, dried tofu, or tempeh, with land or sea vegetables

For Anorexia and Bulimia:

Natto with tamari soy sauce, daikon, ginger, and scallions

Beans are high in protein and are a delicious addition to your diet. It is important not to overeat beans, to chew them very well, and to cook them thoroughly, otherwise they can cause gas, intestinal problems, and a sluggish condition. Beans should always be a side dish, not compromising more than 15 percent of the meal. As they make a heavier dish, beans are more appropriate for supper, somewhat less often for lunch, and generally not for breakfast.

Azuki beans, chick-peas, lentils, and black soybeans are the most yang beans and the best ones to use on a regular basis. Use these beans, and/or bean products such as tofu and tempeh, about three to six times a week (but in small quantities) when healing. Other beans such as pintos, kidneys, black beans, and red lentils can be eaten occasionally, about once a week or less during the healing process, or may be avoided altogether for several months. Soybeans (which are full of protein) need particular attention so that they are cooked thoroughly. They are delicious in combination with vegetables. They can also be eaten in the form of tofu, tempeh, natto, miso, and tamari soy sauce.

Store beans in an airtight container, like a glass jar, in a cool, dry place.

When washing beans, first spread them out a little at a time and remove any stones or anything else that may be mixed in. Then place the beans in a bowl, submerge them in water, and stir. Rinse off any dust that may rise to the surface. Repeat this about 3 times, or until the water becomes clear. As you lift the beans out of the water into a strainer or colander to drain, leave out any heavy dust or residue that remains in the bottom of the bowl.

Except for red and green lentils, beans may be soaked for a few hours or overnight prior to cooking. This softens them and helps to cook them quicker. Azuki beans need only a few hours of soaking and from time to time you may cook them without it, particularly when trying to strengthen an overly yin condition. Soaking is preferred for pinto and kidney beans for more digestibility. Chick-peas and soybeans always need to be soaked, as they are so tough. Use the soaking water when cooking.

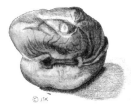

Fig. 22 Chick-pea

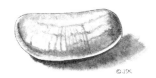

Fig. 23 Baby Lima Bean
(For Occasional Use)

Salt is to be added towards the end of the cooking process, after the beans have already softened, otherwise they will remain hard for a long time. Placing a piece of kombu on the bottom of the pot also helps to soften them while also adding more minerals and flavor. There are three main ways to cook beans.

1. *Boiling:*   This is the method I prefer the most as it cooks the beans gently, slowly, and thoroughly. Beans turn out really delicious and much sweeter when boiled.

    Soak the beans for a few hours or overnight (not necessary for lentils and split peas). Place an optional piece of kombu on the bottom of a pot, then your choice of optional vegetables and finally the beans on top. Add enough water to just cover the beans. Place a drop top inside the pot to sit directly on the beans. This top should be loose fitting to let steam escape on the sides but large enough to cover the inside of the pot as much as possible.

    As the beans expand, slowly and gently pour more *cold* water down the sides of the pot from time to time, always enough to just cover them. The sudden cold water helps the beans to soften more quickly. Bring this to a boil over a medium flame. Then, turn the flame to medium-low and let it simmer for

45 minutes to an hour or so, continuing to add cold water once in a while. Watch closely to see when more water is needed to prevent burning. Do not stir or mix at all, letting the cooking go on undisturbed. This makes for a tastier dish.

When the beans are 70 percent done, add salt and/or miso or tamari soy sauce, remove the drop top, and simmer for another 10 to 20 minutes, or until the beans are completely soft, boiling away any excess liquid.

Lentils

> 1 cup dried lentils
> 2–2$\frac{1}{2}$ cups spring water
> 1 cup diced onion
> 1 cup diced carrots
> $\frac{1}{2}$ cup diced celery
> $\frac{1}{4}$ cup diced burdock
> $\frac{1}{4}$ tsp. sea salt, or 1$\frac{1}{2}$ tsps. tamari soy sauce
> Parsley for garnish

Wash the lentils. Make layers of the onions, celery, carrots, and burdock in a pot. Put the lentils on top and add the water. Bring to a boil, reduce the heat to medium-low, and cover. Simmer for 40 to 45 minutes. Season and simmer for another 10 to 15 minutes. Transfer to a serving bowl and garnish with parsley and serve.

2. *Pressure-cooking:* This is the best method for chick-peas as they are extremely hard and tough. Azuki, pinto, and kidney beans can also be pressure-cooked.

Red and green lentils, split peas, and black and white soybeans may clog the pressure gauge of the pressure cooker and cause a possible explosion, so it is best to boil them. In the case of the lentils and split peas, it does not matter much as they soften very quickly anyway. With soybeans, there are three things you can do to make them safer for pressure-cooking.

A. Boil the (presoaked) soybeans and skim off all the foam that rises to the top. When no more foam appears (maybe in a half hour), place them in a pressure cooker and cook till done.

B. Dry-roast the soybeans before pressure-cooking them. Combining black soybeans with rice or another grain, in addition to the roasting, helps even further.

C. Soak black soybeans for several hours or overnight with ⅛ teaspoon of sea salt for every cup of beans. This helps to prevent the skins from coming off and clogging the gauge.

Azuki Beans, Squash, and Kombu
(Gives vitality, strengthens spleen, pancreas, stomach, and digestion.)

1 cup azuki beans
2 cups buttercup or Hokkaido squash
1 strip kombu, 3″–6″
3–4 cups spring water
½–1 tsp. sea salt
***Optional:* miso or tamari soy sauce to taste**

Place kombu in a pot. Then, cut the squash into big chunks and place them inside, followed by the beans and water. Pressure-cook for 45 to 50 minutes after the pressure has come up, placing a heat deflector underneath, and lowering the flame. Then turn off the flame, bring the pressure down, place the beans back on the stove uncovered, add salt and tamari or miso to taste, and simmer for another 5 to 10 minutes or until any excess water has been boiled away.

When squash is not in season, you may use carrots, turnips, rutabagas, parsnips, or onions. Also, other beans may be substituted for the azuki. Serves 6.

3. *Baking:* Baking is a delicious way to cook beans in the winter as it is very hearty.

This method takes the longest time to prepare but the results are well worth the wait. Pintos, kidneys, and soybeans yield well to baking.

To prepare, first place the presoaked beans in a pot on top of the stove, adding 4 to 5 cups of water for every cup of beans. Bring this to a boil, and boil for 15 to 20 minutes to loosen the bean skins.

Then, pour the beans and liquid into a baking pot. (You can place an optional piece of kombu underneath.) Cover, place in the oven, and bake at 350°F., adding more water from time to time as needed. They may be done in about 3 to 4 hours, depending on the type of beans used.

You may add some vegetables halfway through. The salt and/or tamari or miso should be added after the beans have become soft and creamy. After adding the salt, you can take the cover off and let the beans brown a bit. Then, remove from the stove and serve.

Azuki Beans and Lotus Seeds

2 cups soaked azuki beans
1 cup soaked lotus seeds
1 strip kombu, 8″
8 cups spring water
2 pinches sea salt

Bake, following the above directions. If desired, one cup fresh or dried, soaked lotus root, cut into ½-inch rounds, can be added to this dish.

Other bean variations (pressure-cooking or boiling preferable):

1) **Azuki with chestnuts**
2) **Azuki with carrots and onions**
3) **Azuki with parsnips**
4) **Azuki with raisins and/or rice syrup**

Bean Products

While you are healing, it is best not to over consume bean products. Have a small amount 2 to 3 times a week.

1. Tofu or soybean curd comes in two forms, fresh and dried. The fresh tofu available in Oriental shops is usually prepared using a modern, chemicalized curdling agent, so it is best to buy natural tofu curdled with *nigari* (which comes from sea salt). This is available in natural food stores. Dried tofu is more strengthening and can be used regularly by anyone. Fresh tofu is more yin and should be cooked, especially with some sea vegetables, for persons who are recovering from an illness.

   a) *Fresh tofu:* When you buy fresh tofu, open the package and store the tofu in the refrigerator submerged in fresh water (throw out the water it came in). Before you cook with it, very quickly rinse the tofu under the tap.

   Tofu cooks very quickly and can be boiled, steamed, baked or broiled, sautéed or pan-fried. It is actually done as soon as it is hot. It can be prepared in many ways.

   When boiling tofu, cut it into cubes, put it into boiling water and, when it rises to the top, it is finished. Add it to soup towards the end of preparation. For miso soup, put in the tofu just before you add the miso.

To steam tofu, cut it into smaller cubes, and steam until it becomes hot.

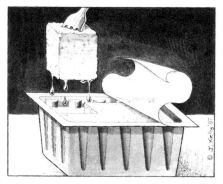

Fig. 24   Tofu

When sautéing with tofu, you do not need to add any extra water as a lot will come out of the tofu. You can press out the excess liquid. To do this, place the whole cube onto a wooden cutting board and prop the board up on one end. Put another cutting board, a heavy plate, or a weight on top of the tofu, and let it drain for one hour.

When pan-frying, baking, or broiling, cut the tofu into slabs, heat a thin layer of oil or water in a skillet or baking/broiling sheet, add the tofu, and cook the slices until they brown or become hot. This only takes a few minutes so be careful not to burn them. Before or after cooking you may spread, dip, or marinate each slice in one of several sauces or dips including: 1) grated ginger and tamari soy sauce, 2) dry-roasted sesame seeds with tamari soy sauce, 3) diluted miso and chopped onions or scallions.

Scrambled Tofu and Corn

> 3 Tbsps. dark sesame or corn oil
> 16 ozs. firm tofu
> 3 cups fresh sweet corn kernels, removed from the cob
> ½–1 tsp. sea salt
> Sliced scallions for garnish

Heat the oil in a pot. Crumble the tofu and add it to the pot. Put the sweet corn on top of the tofu. Cover and cook over low heat for 3 to 4 minutes, or until the tofu becomes hot and the corn is done. Sprinkle a small amount of sea salt on top of the corn. Mix and serve hot. Just before serving, add scallions as a garnish, but, to retain their bright green color, do not cook them.

Variations: The tofu, corn, and scallions may also be sautéed in 2 to 3 tablespoons of water for those who need to limit their oil. Other vegetables may be added or substituted, including cabbage, onions, carrots (cut into matchsticks), and so on. The colors of the vegetables should be bright, and the texture slightly crispy.

Baked Tofu with Miso Sauce

- 1 Tbsp. barley miso
- 2 to 3 tsps. freshly squeezed lemon juice
- $\frac{1}{2}-\frac{1}{3}$ cup spring water
- 16 ozs. firm tofu, sliced into $\frac{1}{2}''$ by 3'' wide slices
- 1 Tbsp. roasted and chopped sesame seeds
- $\frac{1}{4}$ cup sliced scallions or chopped chives

Put the miso and lemon juice in a suribachi. Add the water and puree until the sauce is smooth and creamy. Put the tofu in a shallow baking dish, leaning the slices against one another so they are slightly tilted like this: / / / / / / . Spoon the sauce over the tofu so that the sauce covers the center of each slice. About 1 inch on each side of the tofu slices should be left free of sauce.

Bake the tofu in a preheated 350°F. oven for 15 to 20 minutes. Remove the dish and sprinkle a few sesame seeds and a few scallions or chives on top of the miso sauce. Return to the oven and bake for 2 minutes longer. Remove and serve hot.

b) *Dried tofu:* You can buy dried tofu. It looks like thin, lightly yellow, rectangular wafers. To cook with it, first soak it in water until it softens. Then cut it up into any desired size or leave it whole. This can then be combined with vegetables and treated like one of them. It should be boiled at least 15 minutes. You can also pressure-cook dried tofu and add it to soups and stews. Below is a recipe example.

Pressure-cooked Dried Tofu and Vegetables

1 strip kombu, soaked and cut into squares
1 daikon, cut into large rounds
1 burdock root, cut into large chunks
2 medium onions, quartered
4 shiitake mushrooms, soaked and cut into pieces
1 lotus root, cut into ½″ rounds
6 pieces dried tofu, soaked and cut into strips
1 Tbsp. tamari soy sauce
2 cups spring water

Place kombu in pressure cooker. Place shiitake on top, and the onions around the sides. Add daikon rounds, then lotus root. Add tamari soy sauce and water. Place the tofu on top. Bring to a boil and pressure-cook 15 to 20 minutes. Let pressure come down slowly. Garnish with chopped scallions or parsley. Serves 4 to 6.

3. *Tempeh:* This is a fermented soy product used in Indonesia and now available in many natural food stores. It is energizing and full of protein. Store it in the refrigerator.

You can cook tempeh from a few minutes to 30 minutes or more. The longer that you cook it the more digestible and smooth-tasting it becomes.

In boiling, steaming, pressure-cooking, baking, and sautéing with vegetables, if the tempeh is pan-fried or deep-fried beforehand, it makes the dish extra delicious. It can be deep-fried without any batter or covering. Unlike fresh tofu, add it to your dishes in the beginning of the cooking preparation.

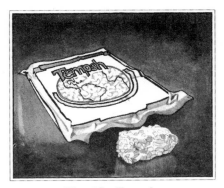

Fig. 25　Tempeh

Tempeh with Sauerkraut and Carrots

1 8-oz. package tempeh
1 cup sauerkraut
2 medium carrots, cut into matchsticks
Spring water
Tamari soy sauce or sea salt to taste
Parsley for garnish

Dry-roast tempeh until slightly browned on both sides, and cut into small squares or triangles. Drain sauerkraut in a colander. Put tempeh in the bottom of a pan and cover with sauerkraut and carrots. Add water to cover tempeh and half of the sauerkraut. Cover and cook approximately 25 minutes.

If you have the greens from the carrots, these can be chopped and added to this dish halfway through the cooking period. Season with tamari soy sauce or sea salt, cook another 3 to 4 minutes, and serve, garnished with fresh parsley.

4. *Natto:* This is a stringy, fermented, soybean product. To some individuals it has an unpleasant smell. However, once a taste is acquired for natto, many people cannot get enough of it.

Natto is rich in protein and vitamin B_{12}; it imparts vitality and is easily digested and assimilated. You can purchase it at natural or Oriental food stores. Natto generally comes frozen; thaw it by leaving it in the refrigerator for a day, or at room temperature for a few hours.

To serve, stir in one or more of the following ingredients: 1) grated daikon, 2) grated ginger, 3) chopped scallions, or 4) diced raw onions with the addition of either tamari soy sauce, umeboshi paste, or sauerkraut. Pieces of nori may also be mixed in. These combinations may be eaten on top of your rice or other grains as a condiment, or in miso soup.

12. Sea Vegetables ━━━━━━━━━━━━━

Sea vegetables are an important and integral part of the macrobiotic diet. They help purify and strengthen the bloodstream, strengthen the intestines, digestive system, liver, pancreas, sexual organs, and enhance mental clarity and awareness. They also help promote beautiful skin and hair. They can be consumed everyday in some form no matter what your condition. They supply calcium, iron, protein, iodine, and vitamins A, B_{12}, and C, as well as various other minerals.

Many people used to (and some still do) cringe at the thought of eating sea vegetables, and considered it an esoteric Oritental food. However, sea vegetables were consumed traditionally by people all over the world including the Celtics, Vikings, Russians, coastal Africans, Mediterranean peoples, North and South American Indians, native Australians, and the early New England settlers (dulse and kombu in their case), as well as people in the Far East. Some varieties may take a while to acquire a taste for, but it is well worth the effort for all the benefits that they bestow.

Sea vegetables are purchased dried (from natural food stores) and can therefore last many years until you use them. They are also easily stored. Any shady, dry place will do.

There are several varieties now available. Kombu is more tough and may take several hours of cooking, unless pressure-cooked, to completely soften. Dulse, on the other hand, can be eaten raw, or like nori, just toasted for a few seconds.

Wash sea vegetables very quickly to retain as much of their nutrients as possible. Submerge hijiki, wakame, and arame in water, rinse off any dust that floats to the top, and lift them out of the water, leaving behind any sand or stones that sit at the bottom. (Arame will probably be pretty clean already as it has been shredded.)

To clean kombu, brush off any dirt or dust with a dry or damp towel. Leave the white-colored substance (which consists of salt and complex sugars) on the surface of the kombu, as it contributes to the flavor and nutritional value. Dulse does not need to be washed in water, but check it very carefully for hidden shells, stones, and tiny fish. Nori and agar-agar should not be washed.

1. *Arame and hijiki:* Arame comes shredded and has a very delicious but mild flavor. Hijiki is naturally stringy and looks like a thicker, darker arame. It also has a richer taste. Hijiki should be soaked

for 3 to 5 minutes until it expands a bit. Remember that it finally becomes 3 to 5 times larger, so be careful not to use more than you need. It is not necessary to soak arame, just quickly rinse it once in cold water.

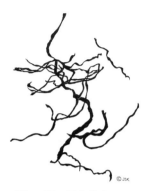

Fig. 26   Dried Arame

Arame and hijiki are cooked the same way, though hijiki takes a longer time, and one can be substituted for the other. They combine really well with root vegetables or with seitan, tofu, tempeh, and fresh corn, as well as other ingredients. They are generally sautéed or just simmered with a small amount of water. It is nice occasionally to sauté the vegetables first before adding the sea vegetable.

Arame with Dried Tofu and Carrots

1 oz. dried arame
2 pieces dried tofu, soaked and cubed
1 tsp. dark sesame oil or water
1 cup carrots, cut into matchsticks
Spring water
2 3 Tbsps. tamari soy sauce
1 Tbsp. mirin

Wash the arame and drain in a colander. Heat the oil or water in a frying pan. Add the arame and carrots and sauté for 1 to 2 minutes. Add the dried tofu, and water to cover the arame and carrots. Add a little tamari soy sauce. Bring to a boil, cover, and reduce the heat to low. Simmer for 40 to 45 minutes. Season with a little more tamari soy sauce and the mirin, and simmer for 10 to 15 minutes longer. When nearly all the liquid has evaporated, mix and serve.

2. *Kombu:* Kombu comes in thick, flat strips which may be anywhere from 3 to 18 inches long. There are recipes throughout this cookbook using kombu, as it enhances the flavor of grains, beans, and vegetable dishes, helping them to soften and/or effectively combining and synthesizing all the ingredients into a whole. It also makes an excellent soup stock. (See *Soup* chapter.) In many cases, kombu is used as an accessory to other ingredients in a dish, but it can be used as a vegetable in its own right. Its texture tends to be tough, so pressure-cooking is often the preferred cooking method, although it can also be boiled.

Kombu needs to be soaked before slicing. It doubles in size, so be careful how much you use. Soak only until it becomes soft enough to cut. Otherwise, it becomes slippery and slicing will be difficult.

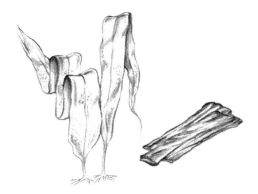

Fig. 27 Kombu

Baked Kombu and Vegetables

1 strip kombu, 3″
2 onions, peeled and quartered
2 carrots, cut into triangular shapes
½ cabbage, sliced into ½″ strips
½ cup spring water
1½ Tbsps. tamari soy sauce

Wash and soak the kombu and put it in a baking dish. Arrange the onions in one side of the dish, the carrots in the center, and the cabbage at the other side, being sure to keep the vegetables separated. Pour the water into a dish and add the tamari soy sauce. Cover and bake in a preheated 375°F. oven for 30 to 40 minutes, or until all the ingredients are tender.

3. *Wakame:* Wakame is a thin, leafy type of sea vegetable, and cooks quickly. You can use it in any recipe that calls for kombu. As is kombu, it is excellent in grain, bean, vegetable dishes, and soups.

Wakame should also be soaked before you slice it. If the soaking water is a bit salty, you can save it for soups, grains or bean dishes where it will be more diluted. Or if you want to use some of the flavor that went into the liquid for your wakame dish, combine a portion of it with fresh water.

The vein portion takes a longer time to cook. Slice that part fairly thin so that it will be finished when the softer leafy sections (which should be sliced into larger pieces) are.

Look under *Vegetables,* *Soups,* and *Condiments* for more wakame recipes.

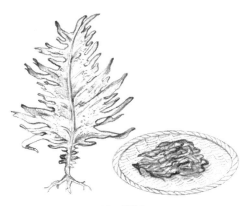

Fig. 28   Wakame

Wakame with Sour-Tofu Dressing

1½ ozs. dried wakame
Spring water
3 umeboshi plums
16 ozs. tofu
¼ cup sliced scallions or chives, for garnish

Wash and soak the wakame. Pour a small amount of water into a pot and bring to a boil. Add the wakame and boil for 3 to 5 minutes. If the wakame is very tender, just dip it in boiling water and remove. After cooking, slice the wakame into small pieces and place in a serving dish.

In a suribachi, puree the umeboshi into a smooth paste. Add the tofu and puree until creamy. Place the dressing in a serving dish and garnish with the sliced scallions or chives. Place a spoonful of tofu dressing on top of each serving of wakame.

4. *Nori:* Nori comes in thin, flat, paper-like sheets. No washing, soaking, or cooking is required except to lightly toast it over an open flame for a few seconds. In Japan, it is used to garnish noodles, grains, and vegetables, and serves as a wrapping for sushi, rice balls, and other items.

After toasting the sheets, you can leave them whole (as you would when you make sushi rolls) or cut them up with your fingers or scissors into any size pieces that you desire. Very small pieces or slivers make a good decorative garnish on top of noodles, grains, vegetables, and so on. One-eighth of a sheet is a nice size for covering and picking up small pieces of grains or vegetables. Two pieces (a quarter of a sheet each) are used to wrap a rice ball.

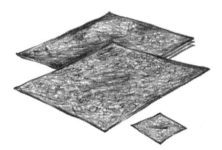

Fig. 29   Nori

Norimaki (Sushi)
(They are handy as appetizers, snacks, and for traveling, and have a very decorative appearance.)

1½ cups cooked short-grain (sticks best) brown rice
1 sheet nori
1 carrot, cut into several lengthwise strips
2–3 uncut (except for the roots) scallions
1″ boiling water in a pot
¼–½ tsp. umeboshi paste
1 pinch sea salt

Add a pinch of salt (for brighter vegetable colors) to the pot of boiling water, and boil the carrot strips until they are soft.

Take the strips out and let them drain. Then, boil the scallions (cut off the roots) for just a second, but not until they loose the bright green color, take them out, and let them drain as well.

Meanwhile, toast a sheet of nori by passing it several times over an open flame (on the dull side only for easier rolling) until it is green but not so much that it is overly crisp and crinkly.

Place a sushi mat onto a cutting board and the sheet of nori on top of it. The halfway fold of the nori should be horizontal from you. Wet your hands and evenly press a 1/4-inch layer of rice onto the nori, leaving 1/2 to 3/4 inch of the top edge (the side away from you) and 1/4 inch of the bottom edge uncovered. Then, make a horizontal indentation in the rice 1 inch up from the bottom of the nori, and spread the umeboshi paste inside the length of it. Then press 1 to 3 carrot strips and the scallions (again horizontally) on top of the paste.

Next, slowly roll the mat and its contents upwards, pressing firmly upon the rice and other ingredients. Try to tuck the vegetables underneath as you keep rolling. Wet the top edge of the uncovered nori (to help in sealing), and complete the roll.

Wash and dry your hands. Place the roll with the sealed edge underneath, wet a vegetable knife (to prevent the rice from sticking to it for smooth, easy cutting), and slowly, carefully but firmly cut the roll into 1-inch slices. Place the slices onto a plate with the inside turned upwards to show their beautiful design, decorate, and serve. Serves 5 pieces.

5. *Dulse:* Dulse can be added raw or slightly toasted to soups, salads, and vegetable, grain, and bean dishes, at the very end of preparation, for extra flavor. It can also be lightly toasted by itself, crumbled and used as a condiment.

6. *Agar-agar:* Agar-agar is used as a jelling agent for kantens and aspics. You can purchase it in the form of bars or powder with the instructions enclosed. (See *Desserts* chapter for kanten recipes.)

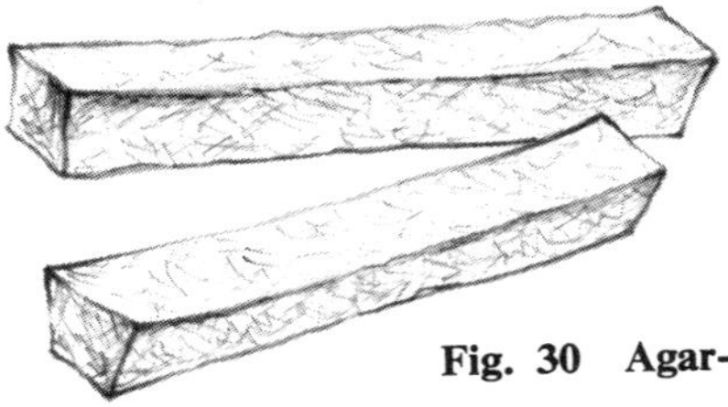

Fig. 30 Agar-agar

13. Seasonings, Condiments, Sauces, and Dressing

Besides your foods and cooking methods, seasonings and condiments play a vital part in the balancing of a meal. As with any other aspect of preparing foods, care must be taken to have enough variety. The chart below is a listing of some of the condiments mentioned in this book. They are categorized into the five tastes. Making sure that you use items from each column insures a well-rounded diet. Some items fit into more than one category. (Do not over use them, especially the salty items. In most cases, just a light accent is enough.)

SOUR	BITTER	SWEET	PUNGENT	SALTY
Pickles	Gomashio	Miso	Ginger	Miso
Sauerkraut	Tekka	Amazake	Scallions	Gomashio
Umeboshi	Green nori	Applesauce	Onions	Umeboshi
Shiso leaves	Parsley	Rice syrup	Grated daikon	Shiso leaves
Rice vinegar	Dandelion	Barley malt	Watercress	Shio kombu
Lemon	Wakame powder	Mirin		Wakame
	Mustard greens	Raisins		powder
	(pickled)			Tamari
				soy sauce
				Tekka

Seasonings:

1. *Sea salt:* Salt is one of the building blocks of life and we cannot survive without it. It is one of the basic ingredients of our blood and gives us vitality, strength, and mental clarity. Learning how to adjust salt intake and finding its balance with oil and water is an important part of mastering the art of cooking.

   Only use white unrefined sea salt. In commercial table salt, much of the valuable trace minerals have been removed. Sugar (dextrose), magnesium and sodium carbonate, and potassium iodine has been added in their place. Such salt depletes important minerals from our body as well as contributing to high blood pressure, heart problems, kidney disorders, and illness in general. Grey sea salt is also not recommended as it can cause excessive tightness in the body.

The amount of salt that we can take depends on our individual condition, our age, our activities, and our environment. Physically active people, adults, persons with a more vegetarian-based history, and persons that live in a more wet, humid, and cold climate can take more salt. (Babies should not take salt at all. It should be gradually introduced to their diet as they grow.) Individuals with a history of heavy meat consumption should carefully limit their intake and may even need to abstain for a short period of time. (These are the persons that benefit from vegetarian, raw food, and salt-free diets, which help to cleanse their bodies. However, after a while, salt and cooked foods should be reintroduced.)

Too much salt can cause hyperactivity, irritability, kidney problems, thirst and anger, among other things. Too little salt can cause poor circulation, mental lethargy, sleepiness, weakness, and so on. (Excess salt can also cause these symptoms at times.)

Your meals should not be overwhelmingly salty. Salt should enhance and draw out the natural flavor and sweetness of your foods, not cover them up. Generally, if you are extremely thirsty or crave fatty, rich foods, or strong yin such as sugar, ice cream, and so on when you finish your meal, it is an indication that too large a dose of salty (or hot) condiments and dishes may have been consumed. Salt is very yang and attracts much yin, so too much makes it difficult to eat in a centered manner.

Plain salt is not recommended for use at the table. (An exception may be a small pinch of it on your fresh fruits to draw out their sweetness.) It is too strong and difficult to assimilate in that form. Various condiments which substitute for salt—such as sea-vegetable powders or a mixture of salt and sesame seeds—are recommended. (See the *Condiments* section in this chapter.)

2. *Miso:* Miso is a paste made from fermented soybeans and sea salt which has been aged for a period of a few months to as much as three years or more. Miso only a few months old is light in color and contains less salt. If older, the color becomes a dark brown, and more salt is needed to keep it going for that long a time.

The darker, longer-time miso is best for healing and is the kind that is assumed when using miso is recommended. The best miso is at least two summers old. There are three basic kinds now available in natural food stores. (Do not buy miso from Oriental food shops. It may be made without using a natural fermenting process, and also may contain chemicals and sugars.)

A. *Hatcho miso:* This is 100 percent soybeans and is the

darkest, most yang variety. It is especially recommended for the cold winter months.

B. *Mugi miso:* This contains barley, is the sweetest of the three, and can be used all year round. It also has medicinal properties.

C. *Genmai (brown rice) or kome (white rice) miso:* These misos contain rice. They are lighter and are good for the summer, though they can also be used year-round. Use this variety less often than the first two.

The short-term miso comes in red, yellow or white. It is sweet, good for the summer, and makes delicious sauces and spreads, but does not have medicinal value.

Buying bulk miso is recommended over the packaged variety, especially when one is trying to heal oneself, as it is more alive. When packing, the miso has to be pasteurized, otherwise it will keep fermenting and may burst the package.

Keep the bulk miso in a cool, dark place, and stir it from time to time. (The short-term kind should be refrigerated.) If a white color starts to appear on the surface, mix it into the bulk of the miso. This substance is a natural bacterial growth and is not harmful. On the contrary, besides adding more minerals and flavor to the miso, it is a reassurance that the miso is organic and alive.

3. *Tamari soy sauce and/or shoyu:* This is a liquid by-product of the miso-making process. It contains fermented soybeans, water, sea salt, and sometimes a small amount of wheat. Be very careful to avoid commercial shoyu as it is artificially aged and is full of chemicals and coloring. To be on the safe side, purchase soy sauce from natural food stores instead of Oriental ones.

Tamari can be added to just about any kind of dish for extra flavor. There are numerous recipes which use it throughout this book.

Like salt and miso, tamari should always be cooked into foods, not added afterwards at the table, as this can make you very tight and disrupt your digestion. Also, be careful that you do not take too much of it.

4. *Umeboshi plum, paste, and vinegar, and shiso-leaf pickle:* Umeboshi plums have very strong medicinal value. They purify the bloodstream, detoxify poisons, stimulate appetite, and at times can help to relieve stomach aches, nausea, and air sickness. (Take them along whenever you travel.) When someone is not feeling

well, we separate the meat of the plums from the pit, grind it into a paste in a suribachi or just chop it very finely and add it to a thick kuzu drink (see *Special Needs* chapter), or serve with rice cream.

Umeboshi plums have been pickled in sea salt and shiso leaves (to give the plums their bright red color) for a year or more. They can be added to just about any dish, and may be used as a substitute for salt, tamari, or miso. One plum is a delicious condiment with a bowl of rice or other grain. (See *Grains and Grain Products* chapter for a rice ball recipe.)

Recently, umeboshi paste and umeboshi vinegar (leftover juice from making these pickles) have become available. They are very handy to cook with and can be added to your dishes. However, they do not have the strong healing qualities of the plum. Therefore, when making *Special Needs* recipes, or when trying to relieve a stomachache (for instance), use the whole plum.

Pickled shiso leaves are also available by themselves. They can be sliced and added to your dishes in addition to, or as a substitute for salt. They are very valuable when dried or baked, and ground into a powder for use as a condiment. In this form, they are helpful for neutralizing strong chemicals in your system.

5. *Oil:* Vegetable oils, which are full of polyunsaturated fatty acids, are needed to build new cells and tissues, to keep warm, for vitamins A and E, to maintain proper metabolism, and to lubricate skin and hair, among other things. However, much of what you need is already found in grains, beans, and seeds, so the intake of extra oil can be kept to a minimum, especially during the initial few months of healing. A healthy person can have a small amount of extra oil nearly everyday in a side dish of vegetables or in a sauce or dressing. Even then, one or two tablespoons are adequate to sauté enough vegetables and grains for a whole family. Also, deep-fried foods should not be consumed more than once a week.

Choose unrefined and cold-pressed oils (meaning that the seeds have been pressed below the boiling point and filtered). Such oils have all their vitamins and nutrients intact, are rich in color, retain the flavor and taste of the original seeds, and are somewhat cloudy in appearance. Please avoid refined oils or oils that have been processed at a high temperature.

Animals oils and fats should be totally avoided as they contain high levels of cholesterol which causes hardening of the arteries and heart disease, among other things.

To digest more oily foods such as fried rice, accompany them with grated ginger, or grated, raw daikon, or plenty of chopped raw scallions.

Keep oils in a tightly sealed container in a cool, dark place, or in the refrigerator.

Sesame oil, especially the dark variety made from roasted seeds, is the most healthy one to use as it is easiest to digest, and is more yang than other varieties. Pumpkin seed oil is an occasional variation, and is also more yang than other oils.

Corn oil (a lighter oil for pastries or pie crusts), safflower, sunflower, and olive oil may all be used occasionally once you are in sound health. It is best to avoid them until then.

6. *Brown Rice Vinegar:*   This is to be used occasionally. It is delicious in sushi, dressings, grain salads, and pickles.

7. *Mirin:*   This is a cooking wine made from sweet rice. It is delicious in sweet-and-sour sauces as well as in beans, vegetables, noodle broths, dressings, and marinades. Use this occasionally; it may be avoided initially for several months.

8. *Ginger:*   Ginger is a hot, pungent, and very delicious root which stimulates the appetite, and activates circulation.

A small amount of grated ginger spices up your grains, vegetables, and noodles. You can extract the juice by squeezing the grated ginger. (The juice is stronger.) Ginger is taken raw or added at the very end of preparations.

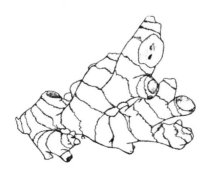

Fig. 31   Ginger Root

9. *Rice syrup and barley malt:* These are the most healthy sweeteners that we use. They are the "honeys" of their respective grains, and are delicious in desserts or cooked in with azuki or black soybeans.

Condiments

Condiments, though we use them sparingly, are an indispensable part of macrobiotic eating. They add one or more of the following to a meal: color, extra variety and flavor, extra vitamins and minerals, appetite stimulation, balance, zest, and in some cases, medicinal value.

A small amount of various condiments may be used everyday to accompany your grains. They allow individuals to adjust their intake of salt, minerals, or oils to fit their own needs. They are easy to overuse so watch out for this, especially when dealing with the saltier varieties such as gomashio or tekka.

Gomashio
(The most commonly used condiment in the macrobiotic diet. It is a perfect balance of salt and oil.)

14–16 Tbsps. black or white sesame seeds
1 Tbsp. sea salt

Dry-roast sea salt in a skillet until it becomes shiny. (Roasting releases moisture in the salt and this helps to make a fluffier gomashio.) Place it into a suribachi, take the pestle and gently grind it until it becomes a fine powder.

Wash and rinse the sesame seeds and drain them in a fine wire-mesh strainer. Place them (they should still be wet) in a skillet and dry-roast them until they pop, emit a nutty fragrance, and can be crushed easily between the thumb and index fingers. Be careful that you do not burn them.

Place the seeds into the suribachi with the salt, and grind them together until the seeds are half crushed and are all coated with salt. Make gentle circular motions using the grooves on the sides of the suribachi. When the gomashio cools off, place it in an airtight glass or ceramic container. (If it is still warm, moisture will collect inside the container and may cause spoilage.) Sprinkle gomashio over your grains and vegetables.

Sesame seeds are high in calcium, protein, iron, phosphorous, vitamin A, and niacin. For variety, add sea vegetable powder or shiso leaf powder instead of salt. (see *Wakame Powder* and *Shiso Leaf Powder* recipes below.)

Shio Kombu

8 long strips (about 12″) kombu
Enough liquid to cover (50% water and 50% tamari soy sauce)

Cut the kombu into 1-inch squares with scissors and soak them in water/tamari for 1 to 2 days. Place them into an uncovered pot, add enough water/tamari to cover, bring to a boil, immediately turn the flame to low, place a heat deflector underneath, and slowly simmer for several hours, until most of the liquid has evaporated. Since this is very strong, have only one or two pieces at a meal.

Nori Condiment

10 sheets nori, broken or cut into small pieces
1 cup spring water
½ Tbsp. tamari soy sauce

Bring all the ingredients to a boil in a small covered pot, turn the flame to low, and slowly simmer for about 20 to 30 minutes, or until most of the liquid has boiled away, leaving a paste of nori.

Kombu-Shiitake Condiment

3 strips kombu, soaked
5 shiitake mushrooms, soaked
½ cup tamari soy sauce
½ cup spring water
1 Tbsp. rice syrup

Slice kombu lengthwise, then into small pieces. Put the kombu in the bottom of a saucepan along with mushrooms, which have been sliced into small pieces. Add tamari soy sauce, water, and rice syrup. Bring to a boil, stir and simmer, covered, until the liquid has evaporated.

Kombu-Sesame Condiment

3 12″ pieces kombu
1 cup sesame seeds, washed and dry-roasted

Brush salt from kombu and place in a baking pan. Bake at 350°F. approximately 10 minutes, or until dark and crisp. Break kombu into small pieces, and grind in a suribachi along with sesame seeds until it forms a powder. Dulse and wakame can also be used in this recipe.

128

Shiso Leaf Powder

Dry-roast 1 cup shiso leaves in a skillet or in the oven at 350°F. until they dry out. Then grind into a powder. This can be combined with seeds, sea vegetable powder, or both.

Sauces and Dressings

It is generally best to use sauces and dressings sparingly. Properly prepared, most good macrobiotic dishes are beautiful and delicious enough to stand on their own. However, they are a nice addition at times, particularly with more bland or lighter dishes, and they can add extra dynamics, as do condiments, without covering up the taste and other qualities of the dish they accompany.

Kuzu Sauce

> 1–1½ cups soup or vegetable stock
> 1 Tbsp. kuzu, dissolved in small amount of water
> Tamari soy sauce to taste
> *Optional:* 2–3 pinches grated ginger

Bring dissolved kuzu and soup stock to a boil, lower the flame, simmer and stir until the kuzu becomes transparent. Add the tamari and ginger, and place this sauce over the grains or vegetables.

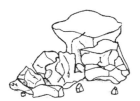

Fig. 32   Kuzu

Red Radishes in Kuzu Sauce

> 1 strip kombu, 3″–6″
> 10 whole red radishes, tops removed
> Spring water
> 3 whole umeboshi plums
> 1 tsp. shiso leaves from the umeboshi plums
> 1–2 Tbsps. diluted kuzu
> Sliced scallions or boiled parsley sprigs for garnish

Put the kombu on the bottom of a pot and add the whole radishes. Add water to almost cover them. Add the whole umeboshi plums, but remove the shiso leaves which the plums were pickled in and save them for salads or pickling. Cook for about 30 to 40 minutes, over low heat. Remove the radishes and put them into a bowl. Strain out the kombu, umeboshi plum pits, and shiso leaves from the cooking liquid. Thicken the liquid with 1 to 2 teaspoons of diluted kuzu and simmer for several minutes. Pour the kuzu sauce over radishes. Garnish with sliced scallions or with sprigs of boiled parsley. Slice the shiso leaves and put them at the side of the bowl with the radishes.

Carrot Tops with Miso
Put the carrot tops and water into a pot. Add the pureed miso in the center of the greens. Cover and cook over low heat for about 5 to 10 minutes, depending on the hardness of the tops. The miso will filter down through the greens.

Garnishes

2 cups finely chopped carrot tops
$\frac{1}{4}$–$\frac{1}{2}$ cup spring water
1 tsp. miso mixed with 3 Tbsps. spring water

To garnish your dishes you can use nori, scallions, parsley, raw onions, sautéed vegetables, red radishes, boiled greens, lemons, grated vegetables, croutons, sliced fruits, roasted seeds and nuts, and so on.

Dressings

Tamari-Vinegar Dressing

Optional: $\frac{1}{4}$–$\frac{1}{2}$ tsp. sesame oil
1 Tbsp. tamari soy sauce
4 Tbsps. brown rice vinegar
1 Tbsp. fresh, grated onion
$\frac{1}{2}$ cup spring water

If using oil, heat it for about 1 minute over a low heat. Puree all the ingredients together in a suribachi and serve.

Scallion-Parsley Dressing

$\frac{1}{2}$ cup sliced scallions

1 Tbsp. chopped parsley
1 cup umeboshi juice (see note below), or 2 umeboshi plums, and
   1 cup spring water
Optional: ½ tsp. sesame oil

Mix ingredients together in a bowl.

Note: Umeboshi juice is made by placing 3 to 4 umeboshi plums in a glass jar, adding 1 cup spring water, shaking, and letting the mixture sit for about 30 minutes. Save plums for another recipe, and use juice in making the dressing.

Miso-Ginger Sauce

1 tsp. barley miso
½ tsp. grated fresh ginger
Spring water

Put the miso in a suribachi and add the grated ginger. Puree with a small amount of water to make a smooth, creamy sauce.

Sour Tofu Dressing

3 umeboshi plums
Spring water
1 cake tofu
¼ cup sliced scallions or chives, for garnish

Put the pitted umeboshi plums in a suribachi and puree to a smooth paste. Add the tofu and puree until smooth and creamy, adding a little spring water to moisten, if necessary. Garnish with sliced scallions or chives. A little tamari soy sauce may be added to this recipe.

For variation:

1) Miso and tamari are interchangeable.
2) Umeboshi is interchangeable with miso and tamari though it does not go well with rice vinegar or lemon.
3) Ginger, onions, parsley, scallions, and chives are interchangeable and can be used singularly or in combination. Using more than two at one time can get a bit too complicated.
4) Lemon can be substituted for rice vinegar.

14. Desserts

You can make delicious desserts using squash, sweet grains, or azuki beans as a base, rather than fruit or flour. The best sweeteners for your health are:

1. Amazake, a drink or a pudding made from fermented sweet rice and a starter called koji, also made out of rice. It can be consumed as it is, as well as being added to other dessert recipes.
2. Rice syrup
3. Barley malt syrup
4. Chestnuts
5. Mirin, a cooking wine made from sweet rice. It is used more in regular cooking than in desserts
6. Raisins and other dried fruits such as apples, peaches, pears, apricots, currants, and cherries
7. Fresh seasonal fruits, cooked
8. Apple juice and cider

Agar-agar and kuzu are natural thickeners you can use in place of eggs, gelatin, and the like.

For more extensive recipes on cookies, cakes, muffins, and so on, refer to other macrobiotic cookbooks. Since this book deals mainly with the healing process, I did not include these less healthful types of desserts.

Amazake
(Also sold ready-made in some natural food stores.)

4 cups sweet brown rice
½ cup koji (sold in some natural food stores)
8 cups water

Soak the rice overnight and pressure-cook for 30 minutes. When done, place it in a glass bowl and, as soon as it becomes cool enough to handle, mix in the koji, cover with a towel, and put it in a warm place. An oven with just the pilot light on, or the radiator, will do. Let this ferment for 4 to 8 hours. Mix it once in a while to help dissolve the koji. The fermentation is done when bubbles start to appear on the surface and when the mixture begins to taste sweet. It becomes sweeter and

sweeter up to a certain point and then it starts to turn sour.
Catch it when it is sweet, place it back into a pot, bring it to
a boil, add a pinch of salt, and turn it off as soon as it starts to
bubble.
You can use the amazake as it is, or you can blend it in
a food mill. For a delicious drink, after you blend it, add
a small amount of water and optional grated ginger, bring to
to a boil, and serve. Or you can let it cool off to make a re-
freshing cold beverage.
To keep the amazake for a longer time, simmer it over a low
flame with a heat deflector underneath until it becomes slightly
brown.

Basic Amazake Pudding

 4 cups amazake drink
 6 Tbsps. kuzu, dissolved in a small amount of water
 2 pinches sea salt
 Optional: ¼ cup raisins

Place all ingredients into a pot, and bring to a boil while stirring constantly with a wooden spoon to avoid lumping and
burning. Then simmer for about 3 minutes, pour into a serving
plate, let it set, garnish, and serve. If it jelled properly, you will
be able to slice it into squares. Serves 8.

Couscous Cake

 2 pints amazake
 2 pints apple juice
 2 pints spring water
 4 cups couscous (dry)
 1 pinch sea salt
 Grated rind of two lemons

Combine all liquid ingredients in a saucepan and bring to a boil.
Add couscous, salt, and lemon rind, and simmer 15 minutes.
Put in an 8-inch cake pan which has been rinsed in cold water.
Bake at 350°F. approximately 15 minutes, or until the cake
begins to come away from the edges of the pan. Cool and top
with apple butter, unsweetened preserves, or fruit glazed with
kuzu.

Chestnut Puree

 2 cups dried chestnuts

5 cups spring water
1 pinch sea salt

Wash chestnuts and dry-roast them in a skillet over low heat for several minutes. Stir constantly to ensure even roasting. Remove and place in a pressure cooker. Add the water and salt, and pressure-cook for about 40 minutes. Mash or grind in a hand food mill until smooth and creamy.

Apple Cider-Lemon Sherbet

2 cups apple cider
2 cups spring water
Juice of 1–2 lemons
2–3 Tbsps. kuzu
1 pinch sea salt

Reserve enough liquid to dilute the kuzu. Bring remaining liquid to a simmer, and add dissolved kuzu. Heat and stir until thickened and smooth. Put into serving bowls. You can add washed grapes or other fruit, such as lightly boiled raisins, strawberries, and so on. Cool and refrigerate.

Rice Syrup-Sesame Seed Kanten

2 cups water
2 cups rice syrup
½ cup sesame seeds
⅓ tsp. sea salt
1 bar agar-agar or 6 Tbsps. agar-agar flakes

Wash, dry-roast, and crush the sesame seeds into a fine powder in a suribachi. Then stir and boil all the ingredients and simmer for 15 minutes. Wet a mold and pour all the ingredients into it. Refrigerate for an hour or so until it jells. Serves 8.

Azuki Kanten

1 cup azuki beans
1½ cups raisins
4 cups spring water
5 Tbsps. agar-agar flakes
3 cups spring water
1 piece kombu, 3″

Soak azuki beans 6 to 8 hours and cook with raisins, kombu,

and 4 cups water in a pressure-cooker for 1 hour. Dissolve agar-agar in remaining 3 cups water, add to the beans, and cook for another 5 minutes. Cool and pour into a serving dish or bowl. This dish can be made with apple juice instead of water, or the water may be sweetened with barley malt.

Strawberry Kanten

2 cups strawberries
4 cups apple juice (or 2 cups juice and 2 cups water)
$\frac{1}{8}$ tsp. sea salt
1 bar agar-agar or 6 Tbsps. agar-agar flakes
1 Tbsp. kuzu diluted in a little cold water

Bring the liquid, salt, agar-agar, and kuzu to a boil, turn the flame to low, simmer and keep stirring until the kuzu becomes transparent and the agar-agar dissolves completely. Add the strawberries. Pour into a serving dish or bowl which has been rinsed with cold water. This dish can be varied by using other dried or fresh fruits and/or nuts. Serves 8.

Pear Marmalade

8 cups sliced pears
$\frac{1}{2}$ cup spring water
1 pinch sea salt

Pressure-cook pears, water, and salt over a low flame 2 to 3 hours. Remove lid and reduce excess liquid by boiling over a low flame, or thicken with kuzu or agar-agar flakes.

Rice Pudding

4 cups cooked brown rice
3 cups apple cider
$\frac{1}{2}$ cup raisins, soaked
Rind of $\frac{1}{2}$ lemon, finely chopped
1 pinch sea salt

Place all ingredients in a pot and bring to a boil. Reduce heat and simmer 30 to 45 minutes. Garnish with roasted, chopped almonds, or apple chunks cooked with a little water, rice syrup, and grated ginger.

Squash Pudding

1 medium-sized buttercup squash (about $2\frac{1}{2}$–3 lbs.)

1 cup spring water
1 pinch sea salt
¼–½ cup barley malt
1 Tbsp. kuzu
1 cup chopped walnuts

Wash squash and remove skin and seeds. Cut squash into chunks and place in a pot with the water. Add a pinch of sea salt, bring to a boil, reduce heat to medium-low, and cover. Simmer until the squash is soft, about 20 minutes. Puree the squash in a hand food mill until smooth.

Return the pureed squash to the pot and add the barley malt. Simmer for about 5 minutes. Dilute the kuzu in a little water and add it to the pureed squash, stirring constantly to avoid lumping. Simmer for 2 to 3 minutes. Remove from the heat and allow to cool slightly. Pour into serving dishes. Serves 4 to 6.

Fish should be eaten as fresh as possible, preferably the same day it is caught, or at least the same day it is purchased. Choose more yin, slow-moving, soft white-meat fish such as sole, flounder, haddock, carp, and so on, as opposed to more active, red-meat varieties such as tuna, salmon, swordfish, and the like. Temporarily avoid shellfish such as clams, oysters, mussels, shrimp, lobster, and crab.

It may be best for some persons to avoid fish entirely, at least for several months, or until symptoms have improved.

Eat two or three times the regular amount of hard leafy greens when including fish in a meal to help balance its strong yang energies. Grated daikon with a few drops of tamari and a bit of grated ginger will help neutralize any possible toxic side-effects of the fish. A few drops of lemon is helpful and a slice of lemon is a beautiful garnish as well.

Clear Fish Soup

1–2 fillets of sole (or other white-meat fish)
1 cup wakame, soaked and cut into 1″ slices
1 bunch watercress, previously boiled for 1 second
3 shiitake mushrooms, soaked and sliced
5–6 cups kombu stock (add shiitake soaking water)
Tamari soy sauce to taste

Bring wakame, shiitake, and kombu stock to a boil, turn the flame down, and simmer for a few minutes until the wakame and shiitake soften. Cut the fish into 1½- to 2-inch pieces, and add them to the soup with tamari to taste. Simmer for 1 to 2 minutes or until the fish turns white. Ladle the soup into individual serving bowls and garnish with the watercress. Serves 6 to 8.

Koi Koku (Carp Soup)

(This very strong soup increases strength and vitality. In Japan, it is served to mothers who have just given birth. It is delicious in the winter and medicinal for those who have become very weak.)

1 small carp (about 2 lbs.)
Equal volume of thinly shaved burdock

½–1 cup bancha tea twigs and leaves (already used to make tea)
Enough liquid to cover, ⅓ bancha tea and ⅔ water
Grated ginger
Miso to taste, pureed
Clean, 100% cotton cheesecloth

Buy a fresh carp, preferably a live one, and ask the fish seller
to kill it for you. Also ask him to carefully (so as not to break
it) remove the gall bladder and the yellow, bitter thyroid bone.
Leave the rest of the fish intact.

Ask the fish seller to chop the whole fish (bones, head, fins,
and all) into 2- to 3-inch chunks. This is difficult to do at home
unless you have the proper knives. Make a sack out of the
cheesecloth and put the used bancha twigs inside like a tea
bag. This helps to soften the fish bones.

Place all the ingredients (including the sack of twigs), except
the miso, into a pressure cooker. Pressure-cook for 1 hour.
Bring down the pressure, take off the lid, add the ginger and
miso to taste, simmer for 5 minutes, and serve. Garnish with
chopped scallions. Serves 6 to 8.

Baked Scrod with Miso

1 cup barley miso
1 cup white miso
2 Tbsps. saké
½ cup mirin
1½–2 lbs. scrod fillets
Grated daikon

Puree the miso, mirin, and saké together thoroughly in a suribachi. Spread half the marinade over the bottom of a shallow
baking dish. Lay the fish fillets on top of the miso spread. Then
spread the remaining marinade on top. Let sit for 4 to 5 hours.
Remove the fish from the marinade. Put the marinated fish
in a baking dish and bake in a preheated 475°F. oven for 15
to 20 minutes. Serve with grated daikon.

Ginger-Broiled Fish Fillets

3 lbs. fresh haddock or other fish fillets
2 Tbsps. tamari soy sauce
2 Tbsps. spring water
1 tsp. freshly grated ginger
Parsley springs for garnish

Place the fillets in a baking dish. Combine the remaining ingredients and pour over the fish. Let sit for approximately 1 hour. Broil the fish for about 5 minutes, or until it is browned on top. If the fillets are very thick, they may need to be turned one time.

Steamed Sole

> **1 medium-sized sole, about 6 ozs.**
> **1 strip kombu, 6″**
> **2 Tbsps. saké**
> **2 shiitake mushrooms, fresh or dried**
> **4–5 broccoli floweretts**
> **Lemon slices for garnish**

Make shallow crosscuts on both sides of the fish with a sharp knife. Soak the kombu for 5 minutes, and put it on the bottom of a small heat-proof ceramic bowl. Put fish on top of the kombu and season with the saké. Nestle the whole shiitake mushrooms next to the fish. If using dried mushrooms, first soak for a few minutes and remove and discard the stems.

Bring about ½ inch of water to a boil in a large kettle. When the steam is up, gently place the ceramic dish containing the sole inside the kettle and cover the kettle. Steam for 10 to 15 minutes. During the last few minutes of cooking, the broccoli can be added, but do not overcook the vegetable.

When the fish is done, remove the ceramic dish from the kettle, and garnish with several slices of lemon. Serve with a dip of tamari soy sauce, water, and grated ginger juice.

16. Beverages ━━━━━━━━━━━━

It is best to drink only when thirsty. Most of us drink out of habit, whether we want to or not (as we often do with eating). If you are always thirsty, some of the dietary reasons may include:

1) Overconsumption of salt
2) Overconsumption of animal products
3) Overconsumption of dry, baked and/or flour products
4) Overconsumption of spices
5) Overconsumption of food in general
6) Not chewing enough
7) Lack of fresh, light dishes
8) Excess of sea vegetables

Good-quality water, such as spring or well water is the best to use. Avoid distilled or highly chemicalized tap water as much as possible.

It is also best to avoid iced or cold drinks (even water), as they can shock and paralyze the digestive system and harden fat accumulations in the body.

The beverages used on a daily basis do not contain caffeine, sugar, carbonation, artificial color, preservatives, stimulants, or alcohol (particularly the hard-liquor varieties). If you are following a more general Standard Diet you can bend this a bit and have small occasional quantities of more yin, good-quality drinks such as green tea, beer, saké, and mint teas. But on a healing diet, these items are best avoided.

The recipes in the *Special Needs* chapter are to be used only when really necessary, and only for a short period of time.

Bancha Twig Tea (Kukicha)
(For daily use, the "brown rice" of beverages.)

1–2 Tbsps. bancha twigs
1½ quarts water

Twig tea generally comes pre-roasted. If not, dry-roast the whole package of twigs and leaves in a skillet for 3 to 4 minutes, stirring gently with a wooden spoon. Take out the 1 to 2 tablespoons that you are going to use and store the rest, after cooling, in an airtight jar.

Add twigs to cold water, bring to a boil, reduce the flame to low, and simmer 10 to 15 minutes, depending on how light or dark you want it. When pouring tea into individual cups, use a bamboo tea strainer (available in natural or Oriental food stores) to strain out the twigs. A regular metal strainer can be used as an alternative. The twigs may be reused several times until they lose their strength, but make fresh tea regularly.

Kukicha contains no caffeine, artificial colorings, or dyes, and is not aromatic. It aids digestion and helps to settle an acidic stomach as it is alkaline in nature. (Most teas are acidic.)

Kukicha or bancha is made from the twigs and leaves of an older, matured tea bush, named *ban* in Japanese. (*Cha* is the Japanese word for tea. Hence, saying "bancha tea" is really saying *ban* tea tea.)

The same bush also supplies some green tea which is made from the topmost and youngest, greenest leaves. This tea is delicious but contains much caffeine and is not recommended for regular use. As the bush becomes older, the caffeine content begins to decrease and finally disappears. Harvesting different sections of the plant, and at different stages in its growth, produces a variety of teas.

Homemade Grain Teas
(Good for daily or regular use.)

To make grain teas, wash, and dry-roast either rice, millet, oats, barley, or wheat, in a dry skillet. Use a wooden spoon to stir. Store what you do not need in an airtight container, after cooling, for later use. Take 2 tablespoons for 1½ to 2 quarts of water, and boil and simmer as in bancha tea.

Mugicha (Roasted Unhulled Barley Tea)
(Good for daily or regular use.)

2 Tbsps. mugicha (available in natural food stores)
1½–2 quarts water

Place the mugicha in cold water, bring it to a boil, reduce the flame to low, and simmer several minutes, the time depending on how strong you want it.

Yannoh/Grain Coffee/Root Coffee
(For more "occasional use.")

4 tsp. yannoh
4 cups water

Bring yannoh and 4 cups of cold water to a boil. Immediately
reduce the flame (as it will boil over), and simmer for several
minutes.
  Yannoh is sold in natural food stores but may be difficult to
find. (When buying grain coffee, make sure that it does not
contain fruits or more yin vegetables such as beets.) You can
make your own homemade yannoh by washing, separately dry-
roasting (till a nutty fragrance is emitted), and grinding the
following:

3 cups brown rice
2½ cups wheat berries
1½ cups azuki beans
2 cups chick-peas
1 cup chicory root

When it is cool, store it in an airtight glass jar. You can experi-
ment and vary different proportions of grains, beans, and vegetables (like burdock or dandelion root) with chicory to find
a winning combination. One hundred percent dandelion-root
coffee can be delicious.

Azuki Bean Tea
(For occasional use, often used medicinally.)

1 cup azuki beans
3–4 cups water
1 piece kombu

Put kombu in the bottom of a pan, then add azuki beans and
water. Boil, reduce the flame to low, and simmer until the
water becomes a rich red. This is good for tight kidneys. Have
one cup a day for 3 days to help loosen them.

Kombu Tea
(For "occasional use.")

1 strip kombu, 6″
2 cups water

Boil the kombu and water until only 1 cup of liquid remains.

Mu Tea
(For "occasional use" only.)

1 teabag Mu tea (sold in natural food stores)
4 cups water

Boil, reduce flame, and simmer for 10 minutes. Mu tea is made of a combination of either 9 or 16 different herbs. The mixture was concocted by my teacher, George Ohsawa, the man who first introduced macrobiotic principles to the Western countries.

Umeboshi Tea
(For "occasional use.")

3–4 umeboshi plums
1½–2 quarts water
Optional: **1–2 shiso leaves**

Separate the meat of the umeboshi from the pits, and tear it into several pieces. Add the *umeboshi* meat and pits to the water, and bring everything to a boil. Turn the flame to low, and simmer for 20 to 30 minutes. This is delicious when cooled in the summer. It also helps to reduce thirst and replaces minerals lost by excessive sweating.

Leftover Vegetable Juice
(For "occasional use.")

You can drink the leftover water from boiling or pressure-cooking vegetables. Just make sure that there is not a lot of concentrated salt in the water.

Vegetable and Fruit Juices
(For "occasional use.")

The juice of any "regular use" vegetable or seasonal fruit on the *Standard Dietary Suggestions* list may be taken once in a while. In the winter it is preferable to heat juice up, especially the yinner fruit juices. They may be helpful occasionally to help relax an overly tight condition.

17. Special Needs ━━━━━━━

You can supplement your meals with home remedies. For more information about their use, read the companion book (*Macrobiotic Health Education Series*), as well as the chapter on *Dietary Adjustments for Obesity and Eating Disorders* in this book. Readers may also consult *Macrobiotic Home Remedies* by Michio Kushi.

Internal remedies: ━━━━━━━━━━━━━

Daikon-Kombu Dish
(To eliminate fat deposits.)

1 strip kombu, 4″
1 daikon root
Spring water
Tamari soy sauce

Soak kombu for 10 minutes. Slice it lengthwise into ¼-inch strips and place them in the bottom of a heavy pot with a heavy lid. Wash daikon and cut it into big chunks. Place a layer of daikon on top of the kombu. Add enough kombu soaking water to just cover the top of the vegetables.

   Cover the pot, bring the water to a boil, lower the flame, and simmer for 30 to 40 minutes, until the kombu is tender. Be careful to make sure the water does not evaporate. Add a small amount of tamari soy sauce, and steam for 2 to 3 minutes more, until any excess liquid is cooked away. This dish may be eaten two or three times per week.

Dried Daikon-Kombu Dish

Follow the above recipe, substituting ½ cup of dried daikon which has been soaked until soft, about 10 minutes. Discard the soaking water in this recipe.

Barley Tea
(To eliminate animal fats from the body.)

¼ cup barley
2½ cups spring water

Wash and dry-roast barley in a heavy skillet for 5 to 10 minutes, stirring constantly. Add water, bring to a boil, lower the flame, and simmer for 15 minutes. Whole wheat berries may also be used for this tea with good results. This drink may be included about three time per week.

Daikon Tea

2 Tbsps. grated daikon
A few drops tamari soy sauce
1 teacup hot bancha tea

Place daikon and tamari soy sauce in a drinking cup, fill the cup with hot bancha tea, stir, and drink. This drink may be used once a day for 2 to 3 days.

Daikon-Carrot Tea

1 Tbsp. grated carrot
1 Tbsp. grated daikon
A few drops tamari soy sauce
1 teacup hot bancha tea

Place the grated carrot and daikon, and the tamari soy sauce in a drinking cup, fill the cup with hot bancha tea, stir, and drink. This drink may be taken once a day for three days.

Black Bean Juice

1 Tbsp. black soybeans
1 quart spring water
Sea salt

Combine washed beans with water. Boil and simmer until only 1 quart of water remains. Add a pinch of sea salt and boil another 5 minutes. Strain. Drink a small cup of this juice 3 times per day to eliminate animal-quality fats and proteins. Drink this several times per week.

Kombu Tea

2 cups water
1 strip kombu, 3″–6″

Bring kombu and water to a boil, reduce the flame to low, and simmer until only 1 cup of water remains. Kombu tea may be taken several times per week.

Tamari Bancha

A few drops tamari soy sauce
1 teacup hot bancha tea

Place of few drops of tamari soy sauce into a teacup. Pour in hot bancha tea, stir, and drink. Use this drink on occasion, as needed.

Ume-Sho-Kuzu
(To strengthen digestion.)

- **1 heaping tsp. kuzu**
- **1 tsp. tamari soy sauce**
- **1 umeboshi plum**
- **⅛ tsp. fresh, grated ginger**
- **1 cup spring water**

Grate the ginger, and chop the meat of the umeboshi plum and put it aside. Dissolve the kuzu in a teaspoon of water until it becomes a liquid, and add it to a small pot with 1 cup of water.

Bring this to a boil, then turn the flame to low as you stir constantly with a wooden spoon. When the mixture becomes transparent, add the tamari soy sauce, umeboshi, and ginger. Drink hot. This drink may be taken on occasion, as needed.

Shiitake Tea
(For eliminating salt and cholesterol.)

- **1 shiitake mushroom**
- **2 cups spring water**
- **1 pinch sea salt**

Soak shiitake for one hour, or until soft. Cut it in quarters, add water, and bring to a boil with a pinch of sea salt. Simmer for about 10 to 20 minutes, or until 1 cup of tea is left. Drink only a half a cup at a time.

This drink may be taken once a day for several days, and periodically thereafter, as required.

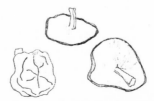

Fig. 33　Dried Shiitake Mushrooms

Ginger Compress
(Helps circulation, dissolves mucus, cysts, tumors, etc.)

6 Tbsps. grated ginger
1 gallon water
Cheesecloth 6″ by 6″
Rubber gloves
3 cotton towels
Optional: **hot plate**
**(A person to give the treatment. It is awkward and not relaxing to
do it yourself.)**

Bring a pot of water to a boil and turn the flame off. Meanwhile, make a sack out of cheesecloth, place the grated ginger inside, and tie the open end into a knot to close it. Immediately after turning off the flame and the bubbles have disappeared, squeeze as much ginger liquid as you can out of the sack and into the pot of water. Then, place the whole bag inside. The point is to put the ginger in as hot a water as possible without boiling it, as boiling would cancel its effectiveness.

Lay the patient down on a bed or some cushions, and let him or her relax. Put on the rubber gloves. Holding the two ends of a cotton towel, dip as much of it as you can into the water. Wring it out and place it on the affected area of the patient's body. If it is too hot, shake it a bit before placing it on. Ideally it should be as hot as one can stand. Cover this with a dry cotton towel to keep it warm for a longer time. Place another towel in the water and when the first towel has cooled off, wring this one out, and exchange it with the first. Again, cover with the dry towel. Continue alternating the towels until the area being treated becomes red. You can reheat (but not boil) the water if it becomes too cool.

The ginger compress is a wonderfully effective home remedy. However, there are situations in which it should be used only as a preliminary to another application, and there are situations where it should not be used at all. Please consult a qualified macrobiotic teacher for guidance. Also, the book, *Macrobiotic Home Remedies* (see bibliography), offers a thorough explanation of this and many other natural remedies.

Buckwheat Plaster
(Draws out excess fluid from swollen areas.)

Buckwheat flour
Enough hot water to form a hard, stiff dough
5%–10% grated ginger
Clean cotton linen

Precede the plaster with a 5-minute application of the ginger compress on the swollen area. Form a dough with the flour, hot water, and ginger, and place a ½-inch layer on the affected area. Cover and tie it on with a strip of linen. Replace the buckwheat every 4 hours. The swelling should go down after several applications or at the most after 2 to 3 days.

Lotus Root Plaster
(Draws out excess mucus, especially from the sinuses, lungs, and bronchi.)

75%–85% grated fresh lotus root
10%–15% pastry flour
5%–10% grated ginger
Cotton linen

Mix these ingredients and spread them ½-inch thick onto a linen cloth. Apply the plaster directly to the skin on the area you are treating. Tie and keep this on for a few hours or overnight, and repeat this for a few days. It is helpful to do a ginger compress on the area before applying the plaster.

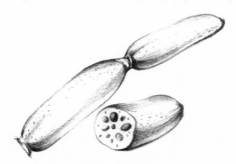

Fig. 34   Lotus Root

Daikon Leaves Hip Bath
(For female sexual-organ troubles.)

4–5 bunches dried daikon leaves
4–5 quarts water
1 handful sea salt
A bathtub of waist-level hot water
A towel

Dry several bunches of fresh daikon tops or greens in the shade until they become dry and brittle. (Use turnip greens if daikon is not available.)

Boil the dried tops with the handful of salt until the 4 to 5 quarts of water turns brown. Straining out the leaves, pour the liquid into the bathtub. The water in the tub (make it hot) should come up to waist level. With a towel covering the upper part of your body, sit in the tub until the whole body becomes warm and begins to sweat (about 10 minutes). Do this for as many days as needed. Follow the bath with a bancha tea douche (see below).

Bancha Tea Douche
(For female sex organs.)

Enough luke-warm bancha tea for douching
½ tsp. sea salt
Juice from half a lemon or equivalent amount of brown rice vinegar

Combine all the ingredients and use as a douche after taking the daikon leaf hip bath.

Salt Pack
(To relieve abdominal pains and cramps.)

Heat 1 to 1½ pounds of white or grey salt in a large skillet, until the salt is very warm. Wrap this salt in a strong, thick cotton towel or bag (such as an old pillowcase). Wrap another towel around it if the pack feels too hot. Apply this pack to the troubled area. Reheat the salt after it has cooled.

Glossary ━━━━━━━━━━━━━━━━━━━━━━━

Agar-agar—A white gelatin made from sea vegetable, used for making *kanten*. You can get it in bars or flakes.

Ame—A natural grain honey derived from rice, barley, or wheat.

Amazake—A sweet porridge or drink made from fermented sweet rice. You can make this at home or buy it in some natural food stores.

Arame—A variety of sea vegetable.

Arepas—Corn cake made from *masa* corn dough.

Arrowroot—A finely ground white flour, used as a thickener, similar to *kuzu* and corn starch.

Azuki beans—Small, red beans. They are good for the kidneys.

Bancha—Tea made from a tea bush which is at least three years old. It helps digestion, and is good for daily use.

Burdock—A long, thin, dark, black root which grows all over the United States, as well as in other parts of the world. It gives one strength and stamina.

Couscous—A partially refined cracked wheat. It is light and cooks quickly. It is good for summer cooking.

Daikon—A long, thick, white root from the radish family. It is pungent when raw and is sweet when cooked. It is an excellent cleanser and purifier of blood, as it helps to break down fat deposits. Grated raw and served with a drop of *tamari* soy sauce, it is a good garnish with oily, greasy foods, making them more digestible.

Dulse—A variety of sea vegetable harvested in Maine, among other places.

Fu—Derived from wheat gluten, you can buy it in natural food stores in either flat, thin sheets, or in round donut shapes. When dry it is like a cracker but when cooked it is more like a noodle. A fun food.

Ginger—A hot, pungent, gnarly-looking, flesh-colored root. It adds zest to your dishes, and also helps circulation whether taken internally or applied externally as in a ginger compress.

Ginger compress—An external treatment made from grated ginger and hot water. It stimulates circulation, and unblocks stagnation (*see recipe*).

Gomashio—A condiment made from roasted sesame seeds and sea salt.

Hijiki—A black stringy variety of sea vegetable.

Hokkaido squash—A delicious squash, similar to buttercup.

Jinenjo—A very hardy, long, flesh-colored, mountain root potato. When grated it becomes a sticky mass and can be eaten with grains, or you can slice it and add it to vegetable dishes. It gives one strength.

Kanten—A gelatin-type food made from agar-agar. It makes a great light dessert when made with fruit and fruit juice. It is also used for aspics.

Kasha—Buckwheat groats.

Kinpira—A thinly sliced or shaved, sautéed-burdock dish, with or without carrots, and seasoned with *tamari* soy sauce.

Koji—Rice which has been innoculated with a form of bacteria. It is used as a starter for making *amazake*, *saké*, *miso*, and *tamari* soy sauce.

Kombu—A long, smooth, flat, thick variety of sea vegetable used in soup stocks, vegetable, bean, and grain dishes, and condiments.

Kukicha—Another name for *bancha*.

Kuzu—A starch made from the root of the *kuzu* plant (called *kudzu* in the United States), which is used as a thickener in vegetables dishes, and for medicinal purposes. When you buy it, it looks like little white rocks.

Lotus root—A tubular, flesh-colored root from the water lily family. It is hollowed out by several lengthwise airholes. It is good for the respiratory system and helps to unclog the sinuses.

Lotus seeds—Seeds of the above. They look like chick-peas.

Masa—A whole corn dough used as a base for *arepas*, *tortillas*, porridges, and so on. You make it at home but some natural food stores have started carrying it already made.

Mirin—A sweet wine made from rice and used in cooking.

Miso—A salty paste made from fermented soybeans with or without grains. Many varieties are available (see *Soups* chapter).

Mochi—Cakes made from pounded sweet rice which are dried and later used in a variety of dishes. It can be made at home or purchased in a natural food store. Make sure to get the brown rice variety instead of the white.

Mugicha—Tea made from roasted barley.

Natto—Stringy, fermented soybeans which when mixed with scallions, *tamari* soy sauce, grated ginger, and *daikon*, makes an excellent companion to a bowl of rice. The taste for it has to be acquired for some people. A good source of protein. It can be homemade or store bought.

Nishime—A method of cooking vegetables with a minimal amount of water.

Nori—A variety of sea vegetable which comes pressed into thin paper-like sheets. It can be used as a garnish, a cover for *sushi* and rice balls, and also as a condiment.

Norimaki—A type of *sushi* which is made by rolling *nori*, rice, and vegetables together into a long roll with a *sushi* mat.

Ohagi—Little balls of cooked, sweet rice which can be covered with seeds, nuts, or *azuki* beans, among other things.

Ojiya—A porridge of soft rice, vegetables, and *miso* (sea salt or *tamari* soy sauce can substituted for the *miso*).

Sea salt—Salt from the sea, much healthier than commercial land salt which contains iodine, sugar, and chemicals.

Seitan—Wheat gluten which has been boiled (and optionally deep-fried as well) with *tamari* soy sauce, *kombu*, and water. It is a good replacement for meat.

Shiitake—A variety of dried mushroom which is helpful in breaking down animal fats within the body. It is used as a soup stock or in vegetable dishes.

Shio kombu—A condiment made from *kombu* and *tamari* soy sauce.

Shiso—Beefsteak plant leaves which are pickled with *umeboshi* plums for added color. It strengthens blood quality, and can be used as a condiment.

Soba—Japanese buckwheat noodles.

Somen—An extremely thin variety of Japanese wheat noodles.

Suribachi—A ceramic bowl with grooves, used with a pestle for grinding and puréeing.

Sushi—Rice formed into little balls and topped with fish or vegetables, as well as rolls (*norimaki*) made from *nori*, rice, and vegetables.

Sushi mat—Bamboo mat used for making *norimaki sushi*.

Takuan—*Daikon* rice-bran pickles.

Tamari—A name given to naturally made soy sauce to differentiate it from the commercially made, chemicalized ones.

Tekka—A strong condiment made out of burdock, carrots, lotus root, ginger, *miso*, and sesame. Available in natural food stores.

Tempeh—Cakes of fermented soybeans, used widely in Indonesia, and available in natural food stores. A good source of protein.

Tofu—A white cake made from soybeans and water, also known as bean curd, available fresh or dried.

Udon—Japanese wheat noodles.

Umeboshi—Salty pickled plums. Helps cleanse the blood and aids digestion.

Wakame—A thin, leafy variety of sea vegetable.

Yannoh—Grain beverage sometimes used as a coffee substitute—made from five different grains.

Bibliography

Macrobiotic Health Education Series

Kushi, Michio. *A Natural Approach: Allergies*. Edited by Mark Mead and John D. Mann. Tokyo: Japan Publications, Inc., 1985.
———. *A Natural Approach: Diabetes and Hypoglycemia*. Edited by John D. Mann. Tokyo: Japan Publications, Inc., 1985.

Macrobiotic Food and Cooking Series

Kushi, Aveline. *Cooking for Health: Allergies*. Edited by Rosalind Rhodes. Tokyo: Japan Publications, Inc., 1985.
———. *Cooking for Health: Diabetes and Hypoglycemia*. Edited by Rosalind Rhodes. Tokyo: Japan Publications, Inc., 1985.

Cookbooks

Aihara, Cornellia. *Macrobiotic Kitchen*. Tokyo: Japan Publications, Inc., 1983.
———. *The Do of Cooking*, Chico. Calif.: George Ohsawa Macrobiotic Foundation, 1972.
Esko, Edward and Wendy. *Macrobiotic Cooking for Everyone*. Tokyo: Japan Publications, Inc., 1980.
Esko, Wendy. *Introducing Macrobiotic Cooking*. Tokyo: Japan Publications, Inc., 1978.
Estella, Mary. *Natural Foods Cookbook: Vegetarian Dairy-free Cuisine*. Tokyo: Japan Publications, Inc., 1985.
Kushi, Aveline. *How to Cook with Miso*. Tokyo: Japan Publications, Inc., 1978.
Kushi, Aveline, with Alex Jack. *Aveline Kushi's Complete Guide to Macrobiotic Cooking for Health, Harmony, and Peace*. N. Y.: Warner Publishing Co., 1984.
Kushi, Aveline, with Wendy Esko. *The Changing Seasons Macrobiotic Cookbook*. Wayne, N. J.: Avery Publishing Group, 1984.
Ohsawa, Lima. *Macrobiotic Cuisine*. Tokyo: Japan Publications, Inc., 1984.

Other Macrobiotic or Related Books

Aihara, Herman. *Basic Macrobiotics*. Tokyo: Japan Publications, Inc., 1985.
Brown, Virginia, with Susan Stayman. *Macrobiotic Miracle: How a Vermont Family Overcame Cancer*. Tokyo: Japan Publications, Inc., 1985.
Dufty, William. *Sugar Blues*. New York: Warner, 1975.
Heidenry, Carolyn. *An Introduction to Macrobiotics: A Beginner's Guide to the Natural Way of Health*. Brookline Mass.: Aladdin Press, 1984.
———. *Making the Transition to a Macrobiotic Diet*. Brookline, Mass.: Aladdin Press, 1984.

154

Ineson, Rev. John. *The Way of Life: Macrobiotics and the Spirit of Christianity.* Tokyo: Japan Publications, Inc., 1985.

Kohler, Jean and Mary Alice. *Healing Miracles from Macrobiotics.* West Nyack, N.Y.: Parker, 1979.

Kotzsch, Ronald E. *Macrobiotics: Yesterday and Today.* Tokyo: Japan Publications, Inc., 1985.

Kushi, Aveline. *Lessons of Day and Night.* Wayne, N. J.: Avery Publishing Group, 1984.

Kushi, Michio. *The Book of Dō-In: Exercise for Physical and Spiritual Development.* Tokyo: Japan Publications, Inc., 1979.

Kushi, Michio. *The Book of Macrobiotics* (Revised edition), Tokyo: Japan Publications, Inc., 1987.

————. *Cancer and Heart Disease: The Macrobiotic Approach to Degenerative Disorders* (Revised edition), Tokyo: Japan Publications, Inc., 1985.

————. *The Era of Humanity.* Edited by Sherman Goldman. Brookline, Mass.: East West Journal, 1980.

————. *How to See Your Health: The Book of Oriental Diagnosis.* Tokyo: Japan Publications, Inc., 1980.

————. *Macrobiotic Home Remedies.* Edited by Marc Van Cauwenberghe. Tokyo: Japan Publications, Inc., 1985.

————. *Natural Healing through Macrobiotics.* Tokyo: Japan Publications, Inc., 1987.

————. *Your Face Never Lies.* Wayne, N.J.: Avery Publishing Group, 1983.

Kushi, Michio and Aveline. *Macrobiotic Pregnancy and Care of the Newborn.* Tokyo: Japan Publications, Inc., 1984.

————. *Macrobiotic Child Care & Family Health.* Tokyo: Japan Publications, Inc., 1986.

Kushi, Michio, with Alex Jack. *The Cancer Prevention Diet.* N. Y.: St. Martin's Press, 1983.

————. *Diet for a Strong Heart: Michio Kushi's Macrobiotic Dietary Guidelines for the Prevention of High Blood Pressure, Heart Attack, and Stroke.* New York: St. Martin's Press, 1985.

Kushi, Michio and the East West Foundation. *Cancer and Heart Disease: The Macrobiotic Approach to Degenerative Disorders.* Edited by Edward Esko. Tokyo: Japan Publications, Inc., 1982.

Mendelsohn, Robert, S. *Confessions of a Medical Heretic.* Chicago: Contemporary Books, 1979.

————. *Male Practice.* Chicago: Contemporary Books, 1980.

Nussbaum, Elaine, *Recovery: From Cancer to Health Through Macrobiotics.* Tokyo: Japan Publications, Inc., 1985.

Ohsawa, George. *Cancer and the Philosophy of the Far East.* Oroville, Calif.: George Ohsawa Macrobiotic Foundation, 1971.

Ohsawa, George, with William, Dufty. *You Are All Sanpaku.* N. Y.: University Books, 1965.

Sattilaro, Anthony, with Tom Monte. *Recalled by Life: The Story of My Recovery from Cancer.* Boston: Houghton-Mifflin, 1982.

Tara, William. *Macrobiotics and Human Behavior*. Tokyo: Japan Publications, Inc., 1985.

Periodicals

East West Journal. Brookline, Massachusetts.
MacroMuse. Rockville, Maryland.
Nutrition Action. Washington, D.C.
The People's Doctor. Evanston, Illinois.

Index